My complete ww program new cookbook for beginners 2024-2025

Walksmart, stay gallant with our best delicious 150+ recipes, to renovate your healthy, + 28day meal plan to balance wellness.

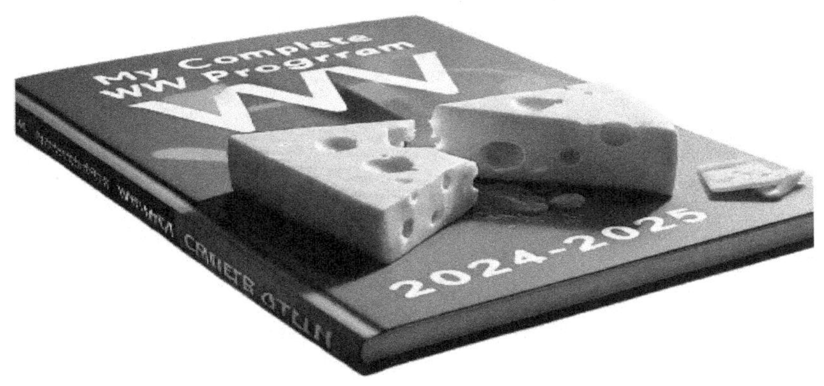

Praise Dogood

TABLE OF CONTENT

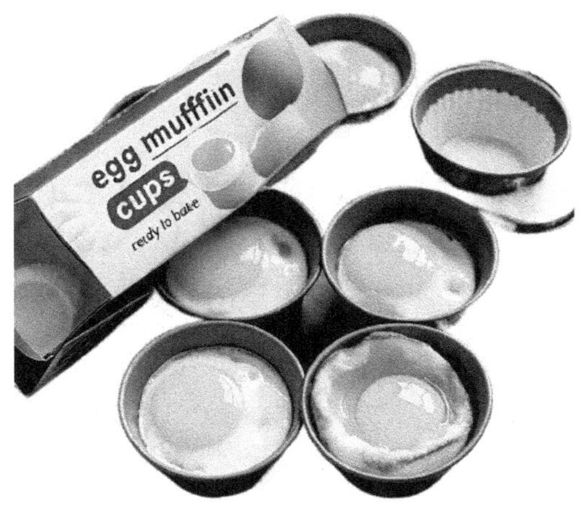

INTRODUCTION

"Welcome to the sweetest weight loss journey of your life! The Weight Watchers Cookbook for Beginners is your ultimate guide to delicious and healthy eating. With 50+ easy and mouth-watering recipes, you'll learn how to cook your way to a happier, healthier you. Say goodbye to bland diet food and hello to flavorful meals that will satisfy your cravings and support your weight loss goals. Let's get cooking and start your journey to a sweet new you!"

This introduction aims to:

- Welcome readers with a warm and inviting tone
- Emphasize the delicious and healthy aspects of the cookbook
- Highlight the ease and accessibility of the recipes
- Encourage readers to start their weight loss journey with the book

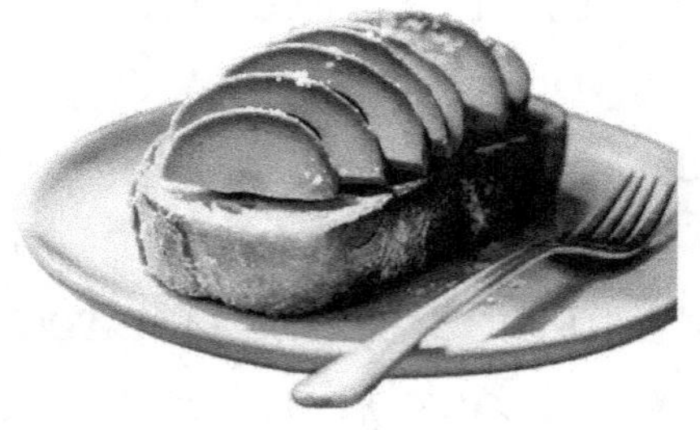

Chapter 1: WHAT IS THE PURPOSE OF WEIGHT WATCHERS?

Weight Watchers is a well-known commercial weight loss program that offers resources and encouragement to anyone who want to cut weight and change their way of living. Since Jean Nidetch started it in the 1960s, it has developed into an all-encompassing system that includes support groups, nutrition education, exercise advice, and a points-based system for monitoring food intake.

The main objective of the Weight Watchers program is to encourage members to make healthier food choices while still allowing for flexibility and enjoyment in their eating habits. This is achieved by assigning point values to items based on their nutritional composition. Members can use their daily and weekly point allotment to schedule their meals and snacks.

To assist members stay accountable and motivated during their weight loss journey, Weight Watchers provides a range of support services in addition to the points system. These services include in-person meetings, online forums, mobile apps, and customized coaching.

Weight Watchers has changed its name to WW over time, emphasizing healthy living and general wellness in addition to weight loss. In order to support people in reaching their health and fitness objectives, the program has been modified to include the most recent findings in behavioral psychology and nutritional science.

Chapter 2: THE ADVANTAGES OF WEIGHT WATCHERS

For those aiming to reduce weight and enhance their general health and well-being, Weight Watchers, or WW, provides a number of advantages:

Flexible and Balanced Approach: WW promotes eating in a balanced way, enabling members to work toward their weight loss objectives while still enjoying a wide range of foods. Members can choose options that best suit their tastes and way of life thanks to the freedom offered by the points system.

Friendly Community: WW offers a friendly atmosphere where members can meet people going through similar experiences through live events, online discussion boards, and social media groups. Maintaining accountability and motivation can be greatly aided by this sense of community.

Education and Resources: WW provides a wealth of information and instructional tools about healthy eating, physical activity, and behavior modification. Members pick up useful techniques for controlling cravings, making better decisions, and getting past barriers to weight loss.

Personalized Coaching: A few WW plans give members access to individualized coaching from qualified experts who may offer direction, accountability, and support based on their own goals and preferences.

Focus on Wellness: WW places a strong emphasis on healthy habits and general wellness in addition to weight loss. The program promotes self-care, mindfulness, and physical exercise as priorities, which enhances participants' emotional and physical well-being.

Accessibility: People with varying schedules, interests, and lifestyles can access WW through mobile apps, online assistance, and in-person meeting alternatives. It is easier for people to join in and continue with the program because of this flexibility.

Long-Term Success: WW wants to assist participants in creating long-lasting, sustainable behaviors. Weight reduction and other health improvements are more likely to be maintained over time when WW emphasizes realistic, slow progress rather than hasty cures.

All things considered, Weight Watchers provides a comprehensive approach to wellbeing and weight loss that takes into account not only what you eat but also how you move, think about health, and consume.

Chapter 3: BREAKFAST RECIPES

Overnight Oats

Ingredients:

- 1/2 cup old-fashioned rolled oats
- 1/2 cup low-fat milk (or non-dairy milk)
- 1/4 cup plain Greek yogurt
- 1 tablespoon chia seeds or ground flaxseed
- 1/2 teaspoon vanilla extract
- Fresh or frozen berries (optional)

Instructions:

1. In a jar or bowl, combine the oats, milk, yogurt, chia seeds, and vanilla extract. Mix well.
2. Cover and refrigerate overnight.
3. In the morning, stir the mixture and top with fresh or frozen berries if desired.

Egg Muffin Cups

Ingredients:

- 6 large eggs
- 1/4 cup low-fat milk
- 1/2 cup chopped spinach or other vegetables
- 1/4 cup shredded low-fat cheese
- Salt and pepper to taste

Instructions:

1. Preheat your oven to 350°F (175°C). Grease a muffin tin with non-stick cooking spray.
2. In a bowl, whisk together the eggs and milk. Season with salt and pepper.

3. Stir in the chopped spinach (or other vegetables) and shredded cheese.
4. Pour the egg mixture into the prepared muffin tin, filling each cup about 3/4 full.
5. Bake for 18-20 minutes, or until the egg muffins are set and lightly golden.

Avocado Toast

Ingredients:

- 2 slices whole-grain bread
- 1 ripe avocado
- 1 teaspoon lemon juice
- Salt and pepper to taste
- Optional toppings: sliced tomatoes, red onion, feta cheese, or Everything Bagel seasoning

Instructions:

1. Toast the bread slices.
2. In a small bowl, mash the avocado with the lemon juice, salt, and pepper.

3. Spread the mashed avocado onto the toasted bread slices.
4. Top with desired toppings, such as sliced tomatoes, red onion, feta cheese, or Everything Bagel seasoning.

Greek Yogurt Parfait

Ingredients:

- 1 cup plain Greek yogurt
- 1/2 cup fresh or frozen berries
- 2 tablespoons low-fat granola
- 1 tablespoon honey or maple syrup (optional)

Instructions:

1. In a parfait glass or bowl, layer half of the Greek yogurt, followed by half of the berries and half of the granola.
2. Repeat the layers with the remaining yogurt, berries, and granola.
3. Drizzle with honey or maple syrup if desired.

Veggie Frittata

Ingredients:

- 6 large eggs
- 1/4 cup low-fat milk or unsweetened almond milk
- 1/2 cup chopped vegetables (e.g., spinach, bell peppers, mushrooms, onions)
- 1/4 cup shredded low-fat cheese
- Salt and pepper to taste

Instructions:

1. Preheat your oven to 350°F (175°C).
2. In a bowl, whisk together the eggs and milk. Season with salt and pepper.
3. Stir in the chopped vegetables and cheese.
4. Pour the mixture into a greased oven-safe skillet or baking dish.
5. Bake for 20-25 minutes, or until the frittata is set and lightly golden on top.

Banana Oatmeal Smoothie

Ingredients:

- 1 ripe banana
- 1/2 cup old-fashioned rolled oats
- 1 cup low-fat milk or non-dairy milk
- 1 tablespoon natural peanut butter or almond butter (optional)
- 1 teaspoon honey or maple syrup (optional)

Instructions:

1. In a blender, combine the banana, oats, milk, and peanut butter or almond butter (if using).
2. Blend until smooth.
3. If desired, add honey or maple syrup for extra sweetness.

Cottage Cheese and Fruit Bowl

Ingredients:

- 1 cup low-fat cottage cheese
- 1 cup fresh berries or diced fruit

- 1 tablespoon sliced almonds or chopped walnuts
- Drizzle of honey or maple syrup (optional)

Instructions:

1. In a bowl, combine the cottage cheese and fresh berries or diced fruit.
2. Top with sliced almonds or chopped walnuts.
3. Drizzle with honey or maple syrup if desired.

Egg and Veggie Muffins

Ingredients:

- 6 large eggs
- 1/2 cup liquid egg whites
- 1 cup chopped vegetables (e.g., spinach, bell peppers, onions, mushrooms)
- 1/4 cup shredded low-fat cheese
- Salt and pepper to taste

Instructions:

1. Preheat your oven to 350°F (175°C). Grease a muffin tin with non-stick cooking spray.
2. In a bowl, whisk together the eggs and egg whites. Season with salt and pepper.
3. Stir in the chopped vegetables and shredded cheese.
4. Pour the egg mixture into the prepared muffin tin, filling each cup about 3/4 full.
5. Bake for 18-20 minutes, or until the muffins are set and lightly golden.

Quinoa Breakfast Bowl

Ingredients:

- 1 cup cooked quinoa
- 1/2 cup low-fat Greek yogurt
- 1/2 cup fresh or frozen berries
- 1 tablespoon sliced almonds or chopped walnuts

- 1 teaspoon honey or maple syrup (optional)

Instructions:

1. In a bowl, combine the cooked quinoa and Greek yogurt.
2. Top with fresh or frozen berries and sliced almonds or chopped walnuts.
3. Drizzle with honey or maple syrup if desired.

Smoked Salmon and Avocado Toast

Ingredients:

- 2 slices whole-grain bread
- 1/2 ripe avocado, mashed
- 2 ounces smoked salmon
- 1 tablespoon diced red onion
- Squeeze of lemon juice
- Salt and pepper to taste

Instructions:

1. Toast the bread slices.

2. Spread the mashed avocado onto the toasted bread slices.
3. Top with smoked salmon, diced red onion, and a squeeze of lemon juice.
4. Season with salt and pepper to taste.

Zucchini Bread Overnight Oats

Ingredients:

- 1/2 cup old-fashioned rolled oats
- 1/2 cup low-fat milk or non-dairy milk
- 1/4 cup grated zucchini
- 1 tablespoon chia seeds or ground flaxseed
- 1 teaspoon cinnamon
- 1/2 teaspoon vanilla extract
- 1 tablespoon chopped walnuts or pecans (optional)

Instructions:

1. In a jar or bowl, combine the oats, milk, grated zucchini, chia seeds, cinnamon, and vanilla extract. Mix well.

2. Cover and refrigerate overnight.
3. In the morning, stir the mixture and top with chopped walnuts or pecans if desired.

Breakfast Burrito Bowl

Ingredients:

- 1/2 cup scrambled egg substitute or liquid egg whites
- 1/4 cup cooked black beans
- 1/4 cup salsa
- 2 tablespoons low-fat shredded cheese
- 1/4 avocado, sliced
- Salt and pepper to taste

Instructions:

1. Scramble the egg substitute or liquid egg whites and season with salt and pepper.
2. In a bowl, layer the scrambled eggs, black beans, salsa, shredded cheese, and avocado slices.

Peanut Butter Banana Smoothie

Ingredients:

- 1 ripe banana
- 1 cup unsweetened almond milk
- 2 tablespoons natural peanut butter
- 1 tablespoon ground flaxseed or chia seeds
- 1/2 teaspoon vanilla extract
- Ice cubes (optional)

Instructions:

1. In a blender, combine the banana, almond milk, peanut butter, flaxseed or chia seeds, and vanilla extract.
2. Blend until smooth. Add ice cubes if you prefer a thicker, colder smoothie.

Veggie-Loaded Breakfast Sandwich

Ingredients:

- 1 whole-grain English muffin or sandwich thin
- 1 egg or 1/4 cup liquid egg whites

- 1/4 cup sautéed spinach or other greens
- 1 slice tomato
- 1 ounce low-fat cheese (optional)

Instructions:

1. Toast the English muffin or sandwich thin.
2. Cook the egg or egg whites as desired (scrambled, fried, or poached).
3. Layer the toasted bread with the cooked egg, sautéed greens, tomato slice, and cheese (if using).

Coconut Chia Pudding

Ingredients:

- 1/4 cup chia seeds
- 1 cup unsweetened coconut milk
- 1 teaspoon vanilla extract
- 1/2 teaspoon ground cinnamon
- Fresh berries or diced fruit for topping

Instructions:

1. In a bowl or jar, combine the chia seeds, coconut milk, vanilla extract, and cinnamon. Stir well.
2. Cover and refrigerate overnight or for at least 4 hours, stirring occasionally, until the chia seeds have absorbed the liquid and formed a pudding-like consistency.
3. Top with fresh berries or diced fruit before serving.

Chapter 4: LUNCH RECIPES

Greek Salad Pita Pockets

Ingredients:

- 4 whole wheat pita breads
- 1 cup cherry tomatoes, halved
- 1 cup cucumber, diced
- 1/2 cup red onion, thinly sliced
- 1/4 cup crumbled feta cheese
- 2 tablespoons olive oil
- 2 tablespoons lemon juice
- 1 teaspoon dried oregano

- Salt and pepper to taste

Instructions:

1. In a bowl, combine the cherry tomatoes, cucumber, red onion, feta cheese, olive oil, lemon juice, oregano, salt, and pepper.
2. Cut each pita bread in half to form a pocket.
3. Stuff each pita pocket with the Greek salad mixture.

Tuna Stuffed Avocado

Ingredients:

- 2 medium avocados
- 1 (5 oz) can tuna, drained
- 1/4 cup diced red onion
- 2 tablespoons lemon juice
- 1 tablespoon olive oil
- Salt and pepper to taste

Instructions:

1. Cut the avocados in half and remove the pits.
2. In a bowl, combine the tuna, red onion, lemon juice, olive oil, salt, and pepper.
3. Spoon the tuna mixture into the avocado halves.

Quinoa and Black Bean Salad

Ingredients:

- 1 cup cooked quinoa
- 1 (15 oz) can black beans, drained and rinsed
- 1 cup diced bell pepper
- 1/2 cup diced red onion
- 1/4 cup chopped fresh cilantro
- 2 tablespoons lime juice
- 1 tablespoon olive oil
- Salt and pepper to taste

Instructions:

1. In a large bowl, combine the cooked quinoa, black beans, bell pepper, red onion, and cilantro.
2. In a small bowl, whisk together the lime juice, olive oil, salt, and pepper.
3. Pour the dressing over the quinoa mixture and toss to combine.

Vegetable Lentil Soup

Ingredients:

- 1 cup dried lentils, rinsed
- 6 cups vegetable broth
- 1 cup diced carrots
- 1 cup diced celery
- 1 cup diced onion
- 2 cloves garlic, minced
- 1 teaspoon dried thyme
- Salt and pepper to taste

Instructions:

1. In a large pot, combine the lentils and vegetable broth. Bring to a boil over high heat.

2. Reduce heat to medium-low, and add the carrots, celery, onion, garlic, and thyme.
3. Simmer for 20-25 minutes, or until the lentils and vegetables are tender.
4. Season with salt and pepper to taste.

Chickpea Salad Sandwich

Ingredients:

- 1 (15 oz) can chickpeas, drained and rinsed
- 1/4 cup diced celery
- 1/4 cup diced red onion
- 2 tablespoons dill pickle relish
- 2 tablespoons mayonnaise
- 1 tablespoon lemon juice
- Salt and pepper to taste
- 4 whole wheat sandwich thins or pita bread

Instructions:

1. In a bowl, mash the chickpeas with a fork or potato masher, leaving some chickpeas whole.
2. Add the celery, red onion, pickle relish, mayonnaise, lemon juice, salt, and pepper. Mix well.
3. Divide the chickpea salad mixture among the sandwich thins or pita bread.

Turkey and Hummus Wrap

Ingredients:

- 4 whole wheat tortillas or wraps
- 1/2 cup hummus
- 8 slices deli turkey
- 1 cup shredded lettuce
- 1/2 cup sliced tomatoes
- 1/4 cup sliced red onion

Instructions:

1. Spread 2 tablespoons of hummus onto each tortilla or wrap.

2. Layer 2 slices of turkey, lettuce, tomatoes, and red onion onto each wrap.

3. Roll up the wraps tightly and slice in half, if desired.

Zucchini Noodle Caprese Salad

Ingredients:

- 2 medium zucchinis, spiralized into noodles
- 1 cup cherry tomatoes, halved
- 1/2 cup fresh mozzarella, diced or torn into small pieces
- 1/4 cup fresh basil leaves, chopped
- 2 tablespoons olive oil
- 2 tablespoons balsamic vinegar
- Salt and pepper to taste

Instructions:

1. In a large bowl, combine the zucchini noodles, cherry tomatoes, mozzarella, and basil.

2. In a small bowl, whisk together the olive oil, balsamic vinegar, salt, and pepper.
3. Pour the dressing over the zucchini noodle mixture and toss gently to combine.

Egg Salad Lettuce Wraps

Ingredients:

- 6 hard-boiled eggs, chopped
- 1/4 cup diced celery
- 2 tablespoons diced red onion
- 2 tablespoons mayonnaise
- 1 teaspoon Dijon mustard
- Salt and pepper to taste
- 8 lettuce leaves (butter, romaine, or iceberg)

Instructions:

1. In a bowl, combine the chopped eggs, celery, red onion, mayonnaise, Dijon mustard, salt, and pepper. Mix well.

2. Spoon the egg salad mixture into the lettuce leaves, dividing it evenly among the leaves.

Grilled Chicken and Veggie Skewers

Ingredients:

- 1 pound boneless, skinless chicken breasts, cut into 1-inch cubes
- 1 bell pepper, cut into 1-inch pieces
- 1 red onion, cut into 1-inch pieces
- 1 zucchini, sliced into 1/2-inch rounds
- 2 tablespoons olive oil
- Salt and pepper to taste

Instructions:

1. Preheat your grill or grill pan to medium-high heat.
2. Thread the chicken, bell pepper, onion, and zucchini onto skewers, alternating the ingredients.
3. Brush the skewers with olive oil and season with salt and pepper.

4. Grill the skewers for 12-15 minutes, turning occasionally, until the chicken is cooked through and the vegetables are tender.

Spinach and Feta Stuffed Portobello Mushrooms

Ingredients:

- 4 large portobello mushroom caps
- 1 cup spinach, chopped
- 1/4 cup crumbled feta cheese
- 2 tablespoons diced red onion
- 2 tablespoons olive oil
- 1 tablespoon lemon juice
- Salt and pepper to taste

Instructions:

1. Preheat oven to 375°F (190°C).
2. Remove the stems from the portobello mushrooms and scoop out the gills to create a cavity.

3. In a bowl, mix together the spinach, feta cheese, red onion, olive oil, lemon juice, salt, and pepper.
4. Stuff the mushroom caps with the spinach and feta mixture.
5. Place the stuffed mushrooms on a baking sheet and bake for 15-20 minutes, or until the mushrooms are tender.

Shrimp and Avocado Salad

Ingredients:

- 1 pound cooked shrimp, peeled and deveined
- 1 avocado, diced
- 1/2 cup diced cucumber
- 1/4 cup diced red onion
- 2 tablespoons fresh cilantro, chopped
- 2 tablespoons lime juice
- 1 tablespoon olive oil
- Salt and pepper to taste

Instructions:

1. In a large bowl, combine the cooked shrimp, avocado, cucumber, red onion, and cilantro.
2. In a small bowl, whisk together the lime juice, olive oil, salt, and pepper.
3. Pour the dressing over the shrimp and avocado mixture and gently toss to combine.

Vegetarian Lentil and Sweet Potato Burgers

Ingredients:

- 1 cup cooked lentils
- 1 small sweet potato, cooked and mashed
- 1/2 cup breadcrumbs
- 1/4 cup diced onion
- 2 cloves garlic, minced
- 1 teaspoon cumin
- 1 teaspoon paprika
- Salt and pepper to taste
- 4 whole wheat buns or lettuce leaves

Instructions:

1. In a bowl, mash the lentils and sweet potato together.
2. Add the breadcrumbs, onion, garlic, cumin, paprika, salt, and pepper. Mix well.
3. Form the mixture into 4 patties.
4. Cook the patties in a non-stick skillet or grill pan over medium heat for 3-4 minutes per side, or until heated through.
5. Serve the patties on whole wheat buns or wrapped in lettuce leaves.

Cauliflower Rice Burrito Bowls

Ingredients:

- 1 head cauliflower, riced
- 1 cup cooked black beans
- 1 cup salsa
- 1/2 cup diced bell pepper
- 1/4 cup diced red onion
- 1/4 cup chopped cilantro
- 1 avocado, diced

- Lime wedges for serving

Instructions:

1. In a skillet, cook the riced cauliflower over medium heat until tender, about 5-7 minutes.
2. In a bowl, combine the cooked cauliflower rice, black beans, salsa, bell pepper, red onion, and cilantro.
3. Top with diced avocado and serve with lime wedges on the side.

Tuna and White Bean Salad

Ingredients:

- 1 (15 oz) can cannellini beans, drained and rinsed
- 1 (5 oz) can tuna, drained
- 1/2 cup diced cucumber
- 1/4 cup diced red onion
- 2 tablespoons lemon juice
- 2 tablespoons olive oil
- Salt and pepper to taste

Instructions:

1. In a bowl, combine the cannellini beans, tuna, cucumber, and red onion.
2. In a small bowl, whisk together the lemon juice, olive oil, salt, and pepper.
3. Pour the dressing over the bean mixture and gently toss to combine.

Vegetable Frittata Muffins

Ingredients:

- 8 eggs
- 1/4 cup milk
- 1 cup diced bell pepper
- 1 cup diced mushrooms
- 1/2 cup diced onion
- 1 cup spinach, chopped
- 1/4 cup grated Parmesan cheese
- Salt and pepper to taste

Instructions:

1. Preheat oven to 375°F (190°C) and grease a 12-cup muffin tin.

2. In a bowl, whisk together the eggs and milk.

3. Add the bell pepper, mushrooms, onion, spinach, Parmesan cheese, salt, and pepper. Mix well.

4. Pour the mixture evenly into the muffin cups.

5. Bake for 20-25 minutes, or until the frittata muffins are set and lightly golden.

Grilled Chicken and Veggie Skewers

Ingredients:

- 1 lb boneless, skinless chicken breasts, cut into 1-inch cubes
- 1 red bell pepper, cut into 1-inch pieces
- 1 yellow squash, sliced into 1/2-inch rounds
- 1 red onion, cut into 1-inch pieces
- 2 tablespoons olive oil
- 1 teaspoon dried oregano

- Salt and pepper to taste

Instructions:

1. Preheat grill or grill pan to medium-high heat.
2. Thread the chicken, bell pepper, squash, and onion onto skewers, alternating the ingredients.
3. Brush the skewers with olive oil and season with oregano, salt, and pepper.
4. Grill the skewers for 12-15 minutes, turning occasionally, until the chicken is cooked through and the vegetables are tender.

Turkey Taco Lettuce Wraps

Ingredients:

- 1 lb lean ground turkey
- 1 packet low-sodium taco seasoning
- 1 cup water
- 8 large lettuce leaves (romaine or iceberg)
- 1 cup diced tomatoes

- 1/2 cup shredded low-fat cheddar cheese
- 2 tablespoons chopped cilantro (optional)

Instructions:

1. In a skillet over medium-high heat, cook the ground turkey until browned and crumbled, about 5-7 minutes.
2. Add the taco seasoning and water, and stir to combine. Simmer for 5 minutes until thickened.
3. Spoon the turkey mixture into the lettuce leaves.
4. Top with diced tomatoes, shredded cheese, and cilantro (if using).

Baked Cod with Lemon and Herbs

Ingredients:

- 4 cod fillets (about 6 oz each)
- 2 tablespoons olive oil
- 1 lemon, sliced
- 2 tablespoons chopped fresh parsley

- 1 tablespoon chopped fresh dill
- Salt and pepper to taste

Instructions:

1. Preheat oven to 400°F (200°C).
2. Place the cod fillets in a baking dish and drizzle with olive oil.
3. Arrange lemon slices over the top of the fish.
4. Sprinkle with parsley, dill, salt, and pepper.
5. Bake for 15-20 minutes, or until the fish flakes easily with a fork.

Quinoa and Black Bean Stuffed Bell Peppers

Ingredients:

- 4 bell peppers (any color), halved lengthwise and seeded
- 1 cup cooked quinoa
- 1 (15 oz) can black beans, drained and rinsed
- 1 cup salsa

- 1/2 cup shredded low-fat cheddar cheese
- 2 tablespoons chopped fresh cilantro

Instructions:

1. Preheat oven to 375°F (190°C).
2. In a bowl, mix together the cooked quinoa, black beans, salsa, and cilantro.
3. Stuff the bell pepper halves with the quinoa mixture.
4. Place the stuffed peppers in a baking dish and bake for 30-35 minutes, or until the peppers are tender.
5. Sprinkle the shredded cheese over the top and bake for an additional 5 minutes, or until the cheese is melted.

Zucchini Noodles with Turkey Meatballs

Ingredients:

- 1 lb lean ground turkey
- 1 egg
- 1/4 cup breadcrumbs

- 1/4 cup grated Parmesan cheese
- 1 teaspoon dried basil
- 1/2 teaspoon garlic powder
- Salt and pepper to taste
- 4 medium zucchini, spiralized into noodles
- 1 cup marinara sauce

Instructions:

1. Preheat oven to 400°F (200°C).
2. In a bowl, mix together the ground turkey, egg, breadcrumbs, Parmesan, basil, garlic powder, salt, and pepper until well combined.
3. Form the mixture into small meatballs, about 1-inch in size.
4. Arrange the meatballs on a baking sheet and bake for 15-18 minutes, or until cooked through.
5. In a skillet, sauté the zucchini noodles for 2-3 minutes, until slightly softened.

6. Add the marinara sauce and cooked
   meatballs to the zucchini noodles and
   toss to combine.

Vegetarian Chili

Ingredients:

- 1 tablespoon olive oil
- 1 onion, diced
- 3 cloves garlic, minced
- 2 bell peppers (any color), diced
- 1 (15 oz) can diced tomatoes
- 1 (15 oz) can kidney beans, drained and rinsed
- 1 (15 oz) can black beans, drained and rinsed
- 1 cup vegetable broth
- 1 tablespoon chili powder
- 1 teaspoon ground cumin
- 1 teaspoon dried oregano
- Salt and pepper to taste

Instructions:

1. Heat the olive oil in a large pot over medium heat.
2. Add the onion and garlic, and sauté for 2-3 minutes until fragrant.
3. Add the bell peppers and continue to sauté for 5 minutes.
4. Stir in the diced tomatoes, kidney beans, black beans, vegetable broth, chili powder, cumin, oregano, salt, and pepper.
5. Bring the mixture to a simmer and cook for 20-25 minutes, stirring occasionally, until thickened.

Baked Salmon with Asparagus

Ingredients:

- 4 salmon fillets (about 6 oz each)
- 1 lb asparagus spears, trimmed
- 2 tablespoons olive oil
- 2 tablespoons lemon juice
- 1 teaspoon dried dill
- Salt and pepper to taste

Instructions:

1. Preheat oven to 400°F (200°C).
2. Place the salmon fillets and asparagus spears on a baking sheet lined with parchment paper or foil.
3. Drizzle with olive oil and lemon juice, and sprinkle with dill, salt, and pepper.
4. Bake for 12-15 minutes, or until the salmon is opaque and flakes easily with a fork, and the asparagus is tender.

Lentil and Sweet Potato Stew

Ingredients:

- 1 tablespoon olive oil
- 1 onion, diced
- 3 cloves garlic, minced
- 2 medium sweet potatoes, peeled and diced
- 1 cup dried lentils, rinsed
- 4 cups vegetable broth
- 1 (14.5 oz) can diced tomatoes
- 1 teaspoon ground cumin

- 1 teaspoon smoked paprika
- Salt and pepper to taste

Instructions:

1. Heat the olive oil in a large pot over medium heat.
2. Add the onion and garlic, and sauté for 2-3 minutes until fragrant.
3. Add the sweet potatoes, lentils, vegetable broth, diced tomatoes, cumin, smoked paprika, salt, and pepper.
4. Bring the mixture to a boil, then reduce heat and simmer for 25-30 minutes, or until the lentils and sweet potatoes are tender, stirring ooccasionally.

Turkey and Vegetable Stir-Fry

Ingredients:

- 1 lb lean ground turkey
- 2 tablespoons low-sodium soy sauce
- 1 tablespoon rice vinegar

- 1 teaspoon sesame oil
- 2 cups broccoli florets
- 1 red bell pepper, sliced
- 1 cup sliced mushrooms
- 1 cup snow peas
- 2 cloves garlic, minced
- 1 teaspoon grated ginger
- Cooked brown rice or quinoa, for serving

Instructions:

1. In a large skillet or wok, cook the ground turkey over medium-high heat until browned and crumbled, about 5-7 minutes.
2. In a small bowl, whisk together the soy sauce, rice vinegar, and sesame oil.
3. Add the broccoli, bell pepper, mushrooms, snow peas, garlic, and ginger to the skillet with the turkey. Stir-fry for 5-7 minutes until the vegetables are tender-crisp.
4. Pour the sauce mixture over the stir-fry and toss to combine.

5. Serve the stir-fry over cooked brown rice or quinoa.

Baked Chicken Fajita Bowls

Ingredients:

- 1 lb boneless, skinless chicken breasts, sliced into strips
- 1 red bell pepper, sliced
- 1 yellow bell pepper, sliced
- 1 onion, sliced
- 2 tablespoons olive oil
- 1 teaspoon chili powder
- 1 teaspoon cumin
- 1/2 teaspoon garlic powder
- Salt and pepper to taste
- Cooked brown rice or cauliflower rice, for serving
- Toppings: shredded lettuce, diced tomatoes, avocado, salsa, etc.

Instructions:

1. Preheat oven to 400°F (200°C).

2. In a large bowl, toss the chicken strips, bell peppers, onion, olive oil, chili powder, cumin, garlic powder, salt, and pepper until well coated.

3. Spread the mixture onto a large baking sheet in a single layer.

4. Bake for 20-25 minutes, or until the chicken is cooked through and the vegetables are tender.

5. Serve the baked fajita mixture over cooked brown rice or cauliflower rice, and top with desired toppings like shredded lettuce, diced tomatoes, avocado, and salsa.

Vegetarian Stuffed Portobello Mushrooms

Ingredients:

- 4 large portobello mushroom caps
- 1 cup cooked quinoa
- 1/2 cup diced tomatoes
- 1/2 cup cooked spinach, chopped
- 1/4 cup crumbled feta cheese

- 2 tablespoons chopped fresh basil
- 2 cloves garlic, minced
- Salt and pepper to taste

Instructions:

1. Preheat oven to 375°F (190°C).
2. Remove the stems from the portobello mushroom caps and scoop out the gills, creating a cavity for the filling.
3. In a bowl, mix together the cooked quinoa, diced tomatoes, spinach, feta cheese, basil, garlic, salt, and pepper.
4. Stuff the mushroom caps with the quinoa mixture, mounding it slightly.
5. Place the stuffed mushrooms on a baking sheet and bake for 20-25 minutes, or until the mushrooms are tender and the filling is heated through.

Shrimp and Broccoli Stir-Fry

Ingredients:

- 1 lb large shrimp, peeled and deveined

- 2 cups broccoli florets
- 1 red bell pepper, sliced
- 2 cloves garlic, minced
- 1 teaspoon grated ginger
- 2 tablespoons low-sodium soy sauce
- 1 tablespoon rice vinegar
- 1 teaspoon sesame oil
- Cooked brown rice or quinoa, for serving

Instructions:

1. In a large skillet or wok, stir-fry the shrimp over high heat for 2-3 minutes until they start to turn pink.
2. Add the broccoli, bell pepper, garlic, and ginger, and continue to stir-fry for 3-4 minutes until the vegetables are tender-crisp.
3. In a small bowl, whisk together the soy sauce, rice vinegar, and sesame oil.
4. Pour the sauce mixture over the stir-fry and toss to combine.

5. Serve the shrimp and vegetable stir-fry over cooked brown rice or quinoa.

Greek Turkey Burgers

Ingredients:

- 1 lb lean ground turkey
- 1/2 cup crumbled feta cheese
- 1/4 cup chopped kalamata olives
- 2 tablespoons chopped fresh parsley
- 1 teaspoon dried oregano
- 1/2 teaspoon garlic powder
- Salt and pepper to taste
- Whole wheat burger buns
- Toppings: sliced tomatoes, red onion, lettuce, tzatziki sauce

Instructions:

1. In a bowl, mix together the ground turkey, feta cheese, olives, parsley, oregano, garlic powder, salt, and pepper until well combined.

2. Form the mixture into patties, about 4-6 burgers.
3. Grill or pan-fry the burgers until cooked through, about 5-7 minutes per side.
4. Serve the burgers on whole wheat buns with desired toppings like sliced tomatoes, red onion, lettuce, and tzatziki sauce.

Chicken and Veggie Foil Packets

Ingredients:

- 4 boneless, skinless chicken breasts
- 2 cups baby potatoes, halved
- 2 cups broccoli florets
- 1 red bell pepper, sliced
- 1 onion, sliced
- 2 tablespoons olive oil
- 1 teaspoon Italian seasoning
- Salt and pepper to taste

Instructions:

1. Preheat oven to 400°F (200°C).

2. Prepare 4 large sheets of foil.
3. Divide the chicken, potatoes, broccoli, bell pepper, and onion among the foil sheets.
4. Drizzle each packet with olive oil and sprinkle with Italian seasoning, salt, and pepper.
5. Seal the foil packets tightly.
6. Place the packets on a baking sheet and bake for 25-30 minutes, or until the chicken is cooked through and the vegetables are tender.

Lentil and Sweet Potato Shepherd's Pie

Ingredients:

- 1 cup dried lentils, rinsed
- 2 cups vegetable broth
- 2 medium sweet potatoes, peeled and diced
- 1 onion, diced
- 2 carrots, diced
- 2 cloves garlic, minced
- 1 teaspoon dried thyme

- Salt and pepper to taste

Instructions:

1. In a saucepan, combine the lentils and vegetable broth. Bring to a boil, then reduce heat and simmer for 20 minutes.
2. In a skillet, sauté the diced sweet potatoes, onion, carrots, garlic, and thyme in a little olive oil or cooking spray until the vegetables are tender, about 10-15 minutes.
3. Add the cooked lentils and their cooking liquid to the skillet with the vegetables. Season with salt and pepper to taste.
4. Transfer the lentil and vegetable mixture to a baking dish.
5. Top with mashed potatoes (or use mashed cauliflower for a lower-carb option).
6. Bake at 375°F (190°C) for 20-25 minutes, or until heated through and the top is golden brown.

Cajun Shrimp and Quinoa Bowls

Ingredients:

- 1 lb large shrimp, peeled and deveined
- 1 tablespoon Cajun seasoning
- 2 cups cooked quinoa
- 1 cup diced bell peppers
- 1/2 cup diced onion
- 2 tablespoons olive oil
- 2 cloves garlic, minced
- Lime wedges, for serving

Instructions:

1. Toss the shrimp with the Cajun seasoning until well coated.
2. In a skillet, heat the olive oil over medium-high heat.
3. Add the bell peppers, onion, and garlic, and sauté for 2-3 minutes.
4. Add the seasoned shrimp and cook for 3-4 minutes until the shrimp is opaque and cooked through.

5. Divide the cooked quinoa into bowls and top with the Cajun shrimp and vegetable mixture.

6. Serve with lime wedges for squeezing over the top.

Grilled Chicken and Vegetable Skewers

Ingredients:

- 1 lb boneless, skinless chicken breasts, cubed
- 1 red bell pepper, cut into chunks
- 1 yellow squash, sliced
- 1 zucchini, sliced
- 1 red onion, cut into chunks
- 2 tbsp olive oil
- 2 tsp dried oregano
- Salt and pepper to taste

Instructions:

1. Preheat grill or grill pan to medium-high heat.
2. In a large bowl, combine chicken, vegetables, olive oil, oregano, salt, and pepper. Toss to coat.
3. Thread chicken and vegetables onto skewers, alternating between ingredients.
4. Grill skewers for about 12-15 minutes, turning occasionally, until chicken is cooked through and vegetables are tender.

Quinoa and Black Bean Salad

Ingredients:

- 1 cup quinoa, cooked according to package instructions
- 1 (15 oz) can black beans, rinsed and drained
- 1 cup corn kernels (fresh or frozen)
- 1 red bell pepper, diced
- 1/4 cup red onion, finely chopped
- 1/4 cup cilantro, chopped

- 2 tbsp lime juice
- 1 tbsp olive oil
- Salt and pepper to taste

Instructions:

1. In a large bowl, combine cooked quinoa, black beans, corn, bell pepper, onion, and cilantro.
2. In a small bowl, whisk together lime juice, olive oil, salt, and pepper.
3. Pour the dressing over the quinoa mixture and toss to combine.
4. Refrigerate for at least 30 minutes before serving to allow flavors to meld.

Baked Salmon with Asparagus

Ingredients:

- 4 (6 oz) salmon fillets
- 1 lb asparagus, trimmed
- 2 tbsp olive oil
- 2 tsp lemon zest
- Salt and pepper to taste

Instructions:

1. Preheat oven to 400°F (200°C).
2. Line a baking sheet with parchment paper or foil.
3. Place salmon fillets and asparagus on the prepared baking sheet.
4. Drizzle with olive oil and sprinkle with lemon zest, salt, and pepper.
5. Bake for 12-15 minutes, or until salmon is cooked through and asparagus is tender.

Turkey and Veggie Lettuce Wraps

Ingredients:

- 1 lb lean ground turkey
- 1 cup shredded carrots
- 1 cup shredded cabbage
- 1/2 cup sliced water chestnuts
- 3 green onions, sliced
- 2 cloves garlic, minced
- 2 tbsp low-sodium soy sauce
- 1 tsp sesame oil

- Lettuce leaves (e.g., Boston, Bibb, or iceberg)

Instructions:

1. In a large skillet, cook the ground turkey over medium-high heat until browned and crumbled. Drain excess fat.
2. Add carrots, cabbage, water chestnuts, green onions, garlic, soy sauce, and sesame oil to the skillet. Cook for 2-3 minutes, stirring frequently, until vegetables are slightly softened.
3. Spoon the turkey mixture into lettuce leaves and wrap them up like tacos.

Zucchini Noodles with Tomato Sauce

Ingredients:

- 4 medium zucchinis, spiralized or julienned into noodles
- 1 (14.5 oz) can diced tomatoes
- 1/2 cup basil leaves, chopped
- 2 cloves garlic, minced

- 1 tbsp olive oil
- Salt and pepper to taste
- Grated Parmesan cheese (optional)

Instructions:

1. In a large skillet, heat olive oil over medium heat.
2. Add garlic and cook for 1 minute, until fragrant.
3. Add diced tomatoes and their juice to the skillet. Season with salt and pepper.
4. Simmer the sauce for 5-7 minutes, until slightly thickened.
5. Add zucchini noodles and basil to the skillet. Toss gently to coat the noodles with the sauce.
6. Cook for 2-3 minutes, just until the zucchini noodles are slightly softened but still retain their crunch.
7. Serve with grated Parmesan cheese, if desired.

Overnight Oats with Berries

Ingredients:

- 1 cup old-fashioned oats
- 1 cup unsweetened almond milk (or milk of your choice)
- 1/2 cup plain Greek yogurt
- 1 tbsp honey (or maple syrup)
- 1 tsp vanilla extract
- 1 cup mixed berries (e.g., blueberries, raspberries, strawberries)

Instructions:

1. In a jar or bowl, combine oats, almond milk, Greek yogurt, honey, and vanilla extract. Stir well.
2. Cover and refrigerate overnight (or at least 4 hours).
3. In the morning, stir the oat mixture and top with fresh berries.

Stuffed Bell Peppers

Ingredients:

- 4 large bell peppers (any color)
- 1 lb lean ground turkey or ground chicken
- 1 cup cooked brown rice
- 1 cup diced tomatoes
- 1/2 cup diced onion
- 2 cloves garlic, minced
- 1 tsp dried oregano
- Salt and pepper to taste

Instructions:

1. Preheat oven to 375°F (190°C).
2. Cut the tops off the bell peppers and remove the seeds and membranes. Place the peppers in a baking dish.
3. In a skillet, cook the ground turkey or chicken over medium heat until browned and crumbled. Drain excess fat.
4. Add the cooked rice, diced tomatoes, onion, garlic, oregano, salt, and pepper to the skillet with the cooked meat. Stir to combine.

5. Stuff the bell peppers with the meat and rice mixture.

6. Bake for 25-30 minutes, or until the peppers are tender.

Vegetable Frittata

Ingredients:

- 8 large eggs
- 1/4 cup milk (or unsweetened almond milk)
- 1 cup sliced mushrooms
- 1 cup diced bell peppers
- 1 cup baby spinach leaves
- 1/4 cup diced onion
- 1 clove garlic, minced
- Salt and pepper to taste
- Cooking spray

Instructions:

1. Preheat oven to 350°F (175°C).

2. In a large bowl, whisk together the eggs and milk. Season with salt and pepper.

3. Spray a large oven-safe skillet with cooking spray and heat over medium heat.
4. Add the mushrooms, bell peppers, spinach, onion, and garlic to the skillet. Cook for 2-3 minutes, until the vegetables are slightly softened.
5. Pour the egg mixture over the vegetables in the skillet.
6. Transfer the skillet to the oven and bake for 15-20 minutes, or until the frittata is set in the middle.

Grilled Shrimp Skewers with Pineapple

Ingredients:

- 1 lb large shrimp, peeled and deveined
- 1 cup pineapple chunks
- 1 red bell pepper, cut into chunks
- 1 red onion, cut into chunks
- 2 tbsp olive oil
- 2 tbsp lime juice
- 1 tsp chili powder
- Salt and pepper to taste

Instructions:

1. Preheat grill or grill pan to medium-high heat.
2. In a large bowl, combine shrimp, pineapple, bell pepper, onion, olive oil, lime juice, chili powder, salt, and pepper. Toss to coat.
3. Thread the shrimp, pineapple, and vegetables onto skewers, alternating between ingredients.
4. Grill the skewers for 8-10 minutes, turning occasionally, until the shrimp are opaque and the vegetables are tetende.

Greek Yogurt Chicken Salad

Ingredients:

- 2 cups cooked and shredded chicken breast
- 1 cup plain Greek yogurt
- 1/2 cup diced cucumber
- 1/4 cup diced red onion
- 2 tbsp fresh dill, chopped

- 1 tbsp lemon juice
- Salt and pepper to taste

Instructions:

1. In a large bowl, combine the shredded chicken, Greek yogurt, cucumber, red onion, dill, lemon juice, salt, and pepper.
2. Mix well until all ingredients are evenly distributed.
3. Serve the chicken salad on top of a bed of lettuce, in a sandwich, or with crackers.

Roasted Sweet Potato and Chickpea Buddha Bowl

Ingredients:

- 2 medium sweet potatoes, peeled and cubed
- 1 (15 oz) can chickpeas, drained and rinsed
- 1 cup cooked quinoa
- 1 avocado, sliced

- 1/4 cup crumbled feta cheese
- 2 tbsp olive oil
- 1 tsp cumin
- Salt and pepper to taste

Instructions:

1. Preheat oven to 400°F (200°C).
2. In a large bowl, toss the cubed sweet potatoes with olive oil, cumin, salt, and pepper.
3. Spread the sweet potatoes on a baking sheet and roast for 25-30 minutes, or until tender.
4. In a large bowl, combine the roasted sweet potatoes, chickpeas, quinoa, avocado slices, and crumbled feta cheese.
5. Drizzle with a little more olive oil or your favorite dressing, if desired.

Lentil and Sweet Potato Soup

Ingredients:

- 1 cup dried lentils

- 2 medium sweet potatoes, peeled and diced
- 1 onion, diced
- 2 cloves garlic, minced
- 4 cups vegetable or chicken broth
- 1 tsp cumin
- 1 tsp paprika
- Salt and pepper to taste

Instructions:

1. In a large pot, combine the lentils, sweet potatoes, onion, garlic, broth, cumin, paprika, salt, and pepper.
2. Bring the mixture to a boil, then reduce the heat and simmer for 20-25 minutes, or until the lentils and sweet potatoes are tender.
3. Use an immersion blender or regular blender to partially puree the soup, leaving some chunks for texture.
4. Adjust seasoning with additional salt and pepper, if needed.

Cauliflower Rice Stir-Fry

Ingredients:

- 1 head cauliflower, riced (or 3 cups cauliflower rice)
- 1 lb boneless, skinless chicken breasts, cubed
- 2 cups mixed vegetables (e.g., broccoli, carrots, bell peppers)
- 2 cloves garlic, minced
- 2 tbsp low-sodium soy sauce
- 1 tbsp sesame oil
- Salt and pepper to taste

Instructions:

1. If using a whole cauliflower, grate or pulse in a food processor to make cauliflower rice.
2. In a large skillet or wok, heat the sesame oil over high heat.
3. Add the chicken and cook for 2-3 minutes until partially cooked.

4. Add the mixed vegetables and garlic to the skillet. Cook for 2-3 minutes, stirring frequently.
5. Add the cauliflower rice and soy sauce. Toss everything together and cook for an additional 5-7 minutes, until the cauliflower rice is tender and the chicken is fully cooked.
6. Season with salt and pepper to taste.

Tuna Stuffed Avocado

Ingredients:

- 2 ripe avocados
- 1 (5 oz) can tuna, drained
- 1/4 cup diced red onion
- 2 tbsp diced tomatoes
- 2 tbsp fresh cilantro, chopped
- 1 tbsp lemon juice
- Salt and pepper to taste

Instructions:

1. Cut the avocados in half lengthwise and remove the pits.

2. In a small bowl, combine the tuna, red onion, diced tomatoes, cilantro, lemon juice, salt, and pepper.

3. Spoon the tuna mixture into the avocado halves, evenly distributing it among the four halves.

4. Serve the stuffed avocados immediately or chill them in the refrigerator until ready to eat.

Baked Cod with Tomato and Basil

Ingredients:

- 4 (6 oz) cod fillets
- 1 pint cherry tomatoes, halved
- 1/4 cup fresh basil leaves, chopped
- 2 cloves garlic, minced
- 2 tbsp olive oil
- Salt and pepper to taste

Instructions:

1. Preheat oven to 400°F (200°C).

2. In a small bowl, combine the cherry tomatoes, basil, garlic, olive oil, salt, and pepper.
3. Place the cod fillets in a baking dish and top with the tomato mixture.
4. Bake for 15-20 minutes, or until the fish is opaque and flakes easily with a fork.

Chapter 7: APPETIZERS AND SNACKS RECIPES

Caprese Skewers

Ingredients:

- Cherry tomatoes
- Fresh basil leaves
- Mini mozzarella balls
- Balsamic glaze Instructions: Thread cherry tomatoes, basil leaves, and mozzarella balls onto skewers. Drizzle with balsamic glaze before serving.

Cucumber Bites

Ingredients:

- English cucumber, sliced
- Fat-free cream cheese
- Everything bagel seasoning

Instructions:

- Spread a thin layer of cream cheese on the cucumber slices and sprinkle with everything bagel seasoning.

Avocado Toast

Ingredients:

- Whole-grain bread
- Ripe avocado
- Lemon juice
- Salt and pepper Instructions: Toast the bread, mash the avocado with lemon juice, salt, and pepper. Spread the avocado mixture on the toast.

Roasted Chickpeas

Ingredients:

- Canned chickpeas, drained and rinsed
- Olive oil spray
- Spices (e.g., cumin, paprika, garlic powder)

Instructions:

Preheat, oven to 400°F (200°C). Pat chickpeas dry and spread them on a baking sheet. Spray with olive oil and sprinkle with spices. Roast for 20-25 minutes, shaking the pan occasionally, until crispy.

Greek Yogurt Dip

Ingredients:

- Plain Greek yogurt
- Cucumber, grated
- Garlic, minced
- Dill, chopped
- Lemon juice

- Salt and pepper

Instructions:

Mix all ingredients together in a bowl. Serve with fresh veggies or whole-grain crackers.

Zucchini Roll-Ups

Ingredients:

- Zucchini, sliced lengthwise into thin strips
- Low-fat cream cheese
- Sundried tomatoes, chopped
- Fresh basil leaves

Instructions:

- Spread a thin layer of cream cheese on each zucchini strip, then sprinkle with sundried tomatoes and basil. Roll up the zucchini and secure with a toothpick.

Baked Parmesan Zucchini Fries

Ingredients:

- Zucchini, cut into fry shapes
- Egg whites
- Panko breadcrumbs
- Grated Parmesan cheese

Instructions:

Preheat oven to 425°F (220°C). Dip zucchini fries in egg whites, then coat with a mixture of panko and Parmesan. Arrange on a baking sheet and bake for 15-20 minutes, flipping halfway, until golden brown.

Deviled Eggs

Ingredients:

- Hard-boiled eggs
- Low-fat mayonnaise
- Dijon mustard
- Paprika
- Salt and pepper

Instructions:

Cut the hard-boiled eggs in half lengthwise. Remove the yolks and mash them with mayonnaise, mustard, and seasonings. Spoon the yolk mixture back into the egg whites and sprinkle with paprika.

Tuna Stuffed Tomatoes

Ingredients:

- Canned tuna, drained
- Low-fat mayonnaise
- Diced celery
- Diced onion
- Salt and pepper
- Cherry tomatoes

Instructions:

Mix tuna, mayonnaise, celery, onion, and seasonings. Cut off the tops of the cherry tomatoes and scoop out the insides. Fill each tomato with the tuna mixture.

Hummus and Veggie Sticks

Ingredients:

- Store-bought or homemade hummus
- Carrots, celery, bell peppers, or other vegetables, cut into sticks

Instructions:

- Serve the hummus with a variety of fresh vegetable sticks for dipping.

Shrimp Cocktail

Ingredients:

- Cooked shrimp
- Cocktail sauce (made with low-fat or fat-free ingredients)

Instructions:

Serve cooked, chilled shrimp with a side of cocktail sauce for dipping.

Bruschetta

Ingredients:

- Whole wheat baguette, sliced
- Diced tomatoes
- Basil leaves, chopped
- Garlic, minced
- Balsamic vinegar
- Olive oil

Instructions:

Toast the baguette slices. Top with a mixture of diced tomatoes, basil, garlic, balsamic vinegar, and a drizzle of olive oil.

Edamame

Ingredients:

- Frozen edamame (boiled or steamed)
- Sea salt

Instructions:

Boil or steam the frozen edamame according to package instructions. Sprinkle with sea salt and enjoy as a protein-packed snack.

Baked Apple Chips

Ingredients:

- Apples, thinly sliced
- Cinnamon
- Cooking spray

Instructions:

Preheat oven to 225°F (105°C). Arrange apple slices on a baking sheet, spritz with cooking spray and sprinkle with cinnamon. Bake for 1-2 hours, flipping halfway, until crisp.

Cucumber Salad

Ingredients:

- Cucumber, sliced
- Red onion, thinly sliced
- Dill, chopped

- White vinegar
- Water
- Salt and pepper

Instructions:

Mix cucumber, onion, dill, vinegar, water, salt, and pepper in a bowl. Refrigerate for at least 30 minutes before serving.

Chapter 8: SIDE DISHES

Roasted Garlic Parmesan Cauliflower:
- Ingredients:
    1. 1 head cauliflower, cut into florets
    2. 2 tablespoons olive oil
    3. 2 cloves garlic, minced
    4. 2 tablespoons grated Parmesan cheese
    5. Salt and pepper to taste
- Instructions:

1. Preheat oven to 400°F (200°C).
2. In a large bowl, toss cauliflower florets with olive oil, minced garlic, Parmesan cheese, salt, and pepper until evenly coated.
3. Spread cauliflower evenly on a baking sheet lined with parchment paper.
4. Roast in the preheated oven for 25-30 minutes, or until cauliflower is tender and golden brown.
5. Serve hot.

Zucchini Noodles with Pesto:
- Ingredients:
  1. 2 medium zucchinis
  2. ¼ cup basil pesto
  3. Salt and pepper to taste
  4. Optional: grated Parmesan cheese for garnish
- Instructions:

1. Using a spiralizer, make zucchini noodles.
2. Heat a skillet over medium heat and add zucchini noodles. Cook for 2-3 minutes until slightly softened.
3. Add basil pesto to the skillet and toss with the zucchini noodles until evenly coated.
4. Season with salt and pepper to taste.
5. Optional: Garnish with grated Parmesan cheese before serving.

Quinoa Salad with Lemon Vinaigrette:

- Ingredients:
    1. 1 cup quinoa, rinsed
    2. 2 cups water or vegetable broth
    3. 1 cup cherry tomatoes, halved

4. ½ cucumber, diced
5. ¼ cup chopped fresh parsley
6. 2 tablespoons lemon juice
7. 1 tablespoon olive oil
8. Salt and pepper to taste

- Instructions:
    1. In a medium saucepan, bring water or vegetable broth to a boil. Add quinoa, reduce heat to low, cover, and simmer for 15-20 minutes, or until quinoa is cooked and liquid is absorbed.
    2. Fluff quinoa with a fork and transfer to a large bowl.
    3. Add cherry tomatoes, cucumber, and chopped parsley to the bowl with quinoa.
    4. In a small bowl, whisk together lemon juice, olive

oil, salt, and pepper to
make the vinaigrette.

5. Pour the vinaigrette over
the quinoa salad and toss
to combine.

6. Serve chilled or at room
temperature.

Grilled Asparagus with Balsamic Glaze:

- Ingredients:
  1. 1 bunch asparagus, trimmed
  2. 1 tablespoon olive oil
  3. Salt and pepper to taste
  4. 2 tablespoons balsamic glaze
- Instructions:
  1. Preheat grill to medium-high heat.
  2. In a large bowl, toss asparagus spears with olive oil, salt, and pepper until evenly coated.

3. Place asparagus spears on the grill and cook for 4-5 minutes, turning occasionally, until tender and lightly charred.
4. Remove asparagus from the grill and transfer to a serving platter.
5. Drizzle balsamic glaze over the grilled asparagus before serving.

Spicy Roasted Sweet Potatoes:

- Ingredients:
  1. 2 medium sweet potatoes, peeled and cut into cubes
  2. 1 tablespoon olive oil
  3. 1 teaspoon chili powder
  4. 1/2 teaspoon paprika
  5. 1/4 teaspoon cayenne pepper (adjust to taste)
  6. Salt to taste
- Instructions:

1. Preheat oven to 400°F (200°C).
2. In a large bowl, toss sweet potato cubes with olive oil, chili powder, paprika, cayenne pepper, and salt until evenly coated.
3. Spread sweet potatoes in a single layer on a baking sheet lined with parchment paper.
4. Roast in the preheated oven for 25-30 minutes, or until sweet potatoes are tender and caramelized, stirring halfway through.
5. Serve hot.

Cucumber Tomato Salad:

- Ingredients:
  1. 2 medium cucumbers, thinly sliced
  2. 1 cup cherry tomatoes, halved

3. 2 tablespoons red onion, finely chopped
4. 2 tablespoons fresh lemon juice
5. 1 tablespoon olive oil
6. 1 tablespoon chopped fresh dill
7. Salt and pepper to taste
- Instructions:
  1. In a large bowl, combine sliced cucumbers, cherry tomatoes, and chopped red onion.
  2. In a small bowl, whisk together lemon juice, olive oil, chopped dill, salt, and pepper to make the dressing.
  3. Pour the dressing over the cucumber and tomato mixture and toss to coat evenly.

4. Refrigerate for at least 30
   minutes before serving to
   allow the flavors to meld.
5. Serve chilled.

Sauteed Garlic Green Beans:

- Ingredients:
  1. 1 pound green beans,
     trimmed
  2. 2 cloves garlic, minced
  3. 1 tablespoon olive oil
  4. Salt and pepper to taste
- Instructions:
  1. Heat olive oil in a large
     skillet over medium heat.
  2. Add minced garlic to the
     skillet and cook for 1
     minute, or until fragrant.
  3. Add green beans to the
     skillet and sauté for 5-7
     minutes, stirring
     occasionally, until green
     beans are tender-crisp.

4. Season with salt and pepper to taste.
5. Remove from heat and transfer to a serving dish.
6. Serve hot.

Mushroom Spinach Quiche Cups:

- Ingredients:
    1. 6 large eggs
    2. 1 cup chopped mushrooms
    3. 1 cup chopped fresh spinach
    4. 1/2 cup diced onion
    5. 1/4 cup shredded low-fat cheese
    6. Salt and pepper to taste
- Instructions:
    1. Preheat oven to 375°F (190°C) and grease a muffin tin.
    2. In a skillet, sauté mushrooms, spinach, and onion until softened.

Remove from heat and let cool slightly.

3. In a large bowl, whisk together eggs, salt, and pepper.
4. Stir in sautéed vegetables and shredded cheese into the egg mixture.
5. Pour the mixture evenly into the prepared muffin tin.
6. Bake in the preheated oven for 20-25 minutes, or until quiche cups are set and lightly golden.
7. Allow to cool for a few minutes before removing from the muffin tin.
8. Serve warm or at room temperature.

Baked Parmesan Zucchini Rounds:

- o Ingredients:

1. 2 medium zucchinis, sliced into rounds
2. 1/4 cup grated Parmesan cheese
3. 1 tablespoon olive oil
4. 1 teaspoon garlic powder
5. Salt and pepper to taste

- Instructions:
    1. Preheat oven to 425°F (220°C) and line a baking sheet with parchment paper.
    2. In a large bowl, toss zucchini rounds with olive oil, garlic powder, salt, and pepper until evenly coated.
    3. Arrange zucchini rounds in a single layer on the prepared baking sheet.
    4. Sprinkle grated Parmesan cheese over the zucchini rounds.
    5. Bake in the preheated oven for 15-20 minutes, or

until zucchini is tender and Parmesan is golden brown.

6. Serve hot.

Cauliflower Rice Stir-Fry:

- Ingredients:
    1. 1 head cauliflower, grated into rice-like pieces
    2. 1 cup mixed vegetables (such as bell peppers, carrots, and peas)
    3. 2 cloves garlic, minced
    4. 2 tablespoons low-sodium soy sauce
    5. 1 tablespoon sesame oil
    6. 1 tablespoon rice vinegar
    7. Salt and pepper to taste
- Instructions:
    1. Heat sesame oil in a large skillet or wok over medium-high heat.

2. Add minced garlic to the skillet and cook for 1 minute, until fragrant.
3. Add mixed vegetables to the skillet and stir-fry for 3-5 minutes, or until tender-crisp.
4. Add cauliflower rice to the skillet and cook for an additional 3-4 minutes, stirring frequently.
5. In a small bowl, whisk together soy sauce and rice vinegar. Pour the mixture over the cauliflower rice and vegetables, tossing to combine.
6. Cook for another 2-3 minutes, or until heated through.
7. Season with salt and pepper to taste.
8. Serve hot.

Greek Cucumber Salad:

- Ingredients:
    1. 2 cucumbers, diced
    2. 1 cup cherry tomatoes, halved
    3. 1/4 cup red onion, thinly sliced
    4. 1/4 cup crumbled feta cheese
    5. 2 tablespoons fresh lemon juice
    6. 1 tablespoon extra virgin olive oil
    7. 1 tablespoon chopped fresh dill
    8. Salt and pepper to taste
- Instructions:
    1. In a large bowl, combine diced cucumbers, cherry tomatoes, sliced red onion, and crumbled feta cheese.
    2. In a small bowl, whisk together lemon juice, olive oil, chopped dill, salt, and

pepper to make the dressing.

3. Pour the dressing over the cucumber salad and toss to coat evenly.
4. Refrigerate for at least 30 minutes before serving to allow the flavors to meld.
5. Serve chilled.

Roasted Brussels Sprouts with Balsamic Glaze:

- Ingredients:
    1. 1 pound Brussels sprouts, trimmed and halved
    2. 2 tablespoons olive oil
    3. Salt and pepper to taste
    4. 2 tablespoons balsamic glaze
- Instructions:
    1. Preheat oven to 400°F (200°C) and line a baking sheet with parchment paper.

2. In a large bowl, toss Brussels sprouts with olive oil, salt, and pepper until evenly coated.
3. Spread Brussels sprouts in a single layer on the prepared baking sheet.
4. Roast in the preheated oven for 25-30 minutes, or until Brussels sprouts are tender and caramelized, stirring halfway through.
5. Drizzle balsamic glaze over the roasted Brussels sprouts before serving.
6. Serve hot.

Mango Avocado Salsa:

- Ingredients:
  1. 1 ripe mango, diced
  2. 1 ripe avocado, diced
  3. 1/4 cup red onion, finely chopped

4. 1/4 cup fresh cilantro, chopped
5. 1 jalapeño pepper, seeded and finely chopped
6. Juice of 1 lime
7. Salt and pepper to taste
- Instructions:
  1. In a medium bowl, combine diced mango, diced avocado, chopped red onion, chopped cilantro, and chopped jalapeño pepper.
  2. Squeeze lime juice over the mixture and gently toss to combine.
  3. Season with salt and pepper to taste.
  4. Serve immediately as a topping for grilled chicken, fish, or as a dip with whole grain tortilla chips.

Lemon Garlic Roasted Broccoli:

- Ingredients:
    1. 1 pound broccoli florets
    2. 2 tablespoons olive oil
    3. 2 cloves garlic, minced
    4. Zest of 1 lemon
    5. Juice of 1/2 lemon
    6. Salt and pepper to taste
- Instructions:
    1. Preheat oven to 425°F (220°C) and line a baking sheet with parchment paper.
    2. In a large bowl, toss broccoli florets with olive oil, minced garlic, lemon zest, lemon juice, salt, and pepper until evenly coated.
    3. Spread broccoli in a single layer on the prepared baking sheet.
    4. Roast in the preheated oven for 20-25 minutes, or until broccoli is tender and

slightly charred, stirring halfway through.
5. Serve hot.

Cauliflower Mashed "Potatoes":

- Ingredients:
    1. 1 medium head cauliflower, cut into florets
    2. 2 cloves garlic, minced
    3. 2 tablespoons low-fat cream cheese
    4. 1 tablespoon unsalted butter
    5. Salt and pepper to taste
    6. Chopped chives for garnish (optional)
- Instructions:
    1. Place cauliflower florets in a steamer basket over boiling water and steam for 10-12 minutes, or until tender.

2. Transfer steamed cauliflower to a food processor.
3. Add minced garlic, low-fat cream cheese, and unsalted butter to the food processor. Process until smooth and creamy.
4. Season with salt and pepper to taste.
5. Garnish with chopped chives, if desired, before serving.

Spinach and Strawberry Salad:

- Ingredients:
    1. 4 cups baby spinach leaves
    2. 1 cup sliced strawberries
    3. 1/4 cup sliced almonds
    4. 2 tablespoons crumbled feta cheese
    5. 2 tablespoons balsamic vinaigrette dressing

(store-bought or homemade)

- ○ Instructions:
    1. In a large bowl, combine baby spinach leaves, sliced strawberries, sliced almonds, and crumbled feta cheese.
    2. Drizzle balsamic vinaigrette dressing over the salad and toss gently to coat evenly.
    3. Serve immediately as a refreshing side dish or light lunch option.

Chapter 9: DESERT

Fruit Salad with Honey Lime Dressing:

- ○ Ingredients:
    1. 2 cups mixed fresh fruits (such as strawberries,

blueberries, grapes, and kiwi), diced

2. 1 tablespoon honey
3. Juice of 1 lime
4. Fresh mint leaves for garnish (optional)

- Instructions:
    1. In a large bowl, combine diced mixed fruits.
    2. In a small bowl, whisk together honey and lime juice to make the dressing.
    3. Pour the dressing over the mixed fruits and toss gently to coat evenly.
    4. Garnish with fresh mint leaves, if desired, before serving.
    5. Serve immediately as a light and refreshing dessert option.

Greek Yogurt Parfait:

- Ingredients:

1. 1 cup non-fat Greek yogurt
2. 1/2 cup mixed berries (such as raspberries, blueberries, and strawberries)
3. 1 tablespoon honey
4. 2 tablespoons granola

- Instructions:
    1. In a serving glass or bowl, layer non-fat Greek yogurt, mixed berries, and granola.
    2. Drizzle honey over the top layer.
    3. Repeat the layers if desired.
    4. Serve immediately as a satisfying and protein-rich dessert option.

Baked Apples with Cinnamon:

- Ingredients:
    1. 2 medium apples, cored

2. 1 tablespoon unsalted butter or coconut oil

3. 1 tablespoon brown sugar or sweetener of choice

4. 1/2 teaspoon ground cinnamon

5. 2 tablespoons chopped nuts (such as walnuts or almonds) (optional)

- Instructions:
    1. Preheat oven to 375°F (190°C).
    2. Place cored apples in a baking dish.
    3. In a small bowl, mix together unsalted butter or coconut oil, brown sugar or sweetener, and ground cinnamon.
    4. Spoon the mixture into the center of each apple.
    5. Bake in the preheated oven for 25-30 minutes, or until apples are tender.

6. Optional: Sprinkle chopped nuts over the baked apples before serving.
7. Serve warm as a comforting and low-calorie dessert option.

Frozen Banana "Ice Cream":

- Ingredients:
    1. 2 ripe bananas, peeled and sliced
    2. 1 tablespoon unsweetened cocoa powder
    3. 1 tablespoon peanut butter or almond butter (optional)
    4. 1 tablespoon chopped nuts (such as almonds or peanuts) (optional)
- Instructions:
    1. Place sliced bananas in a single layer on a

parchment paper-lined baking sheet.

2. Freeze bananas for at least 2 hours or until completely frozen.
3. Transfer frozen banana slices to a blender or food processor.
4. Add unsweetened cocoa powder and peanut butter or almond butter, if using.
5. Blend until smooth and creamy, scraping down the sides as needed.
6. Optional: Stir in chopped nuts for added crunch.
7. Serve immediately as a guilt-free and indulgent-tasting dessert ooption.

Mixed Berry Frozen Yogurt Bark:

- Ingredients:

1. 2 cups non-fat Greek yogurt
2. 1 tablespoon honey or maple syrup
3. 1 cup mixed berries (such as strawberries, blueberries, and raspberries), chopped
4. 2 tablespoons unsweetened shredded coconut (optional)

- Instructions:
    1. Line a baking sheet with parchment paper.
    2. In a bowl, mix together Greek yogurt and honey or maple syrup until well combined.
    3. Spread the yogurt mixture evenly onto the prepared baking sheet.
    4. Sprinkle chopped mixed berries and shredded

coconut evenly over the yogurt.

5. Place the baking sheet in the freezer and freeze for at least 4 hours or until firm.
6. Once frozen, break the yogurt bark into pieces.
7. Serve immediately as a refreshing and guilt-free frozen treat.

Pineapple Coconut Popsicles:

- Ingredients:
    1. 2 cups fresh pineapple chunks
    2. 1 cup light coconut milk
    3. 1 tablespoon honey or maple syrup (optional)
- Instructions:
    1. Place pineapple chunks, coconut milk, and honey or maple syrup (if using) in a blender.

2. Blend until smooth and well combined.

3. Pour the mixture into popsicle molds.

4. Insert popsicle sticks into the molds.

5. Freeze for at least 4 hours or until completely frozen.

6. Once frozen, remove the popsicles from the molds and serve immediately.

Chocolate Covered Strawberries:

- Ingredients:
  1. 12 large strawberries, washed and dried
  2. 2 ounces dark chocolate, chopped
  3. 1 teaspoon coconut oil
- Instructions:
  1. Line a baking sheet with parchment paper.

2. In a microwave-safe bowl, combine chopped dark chocolate and coconut oil.
3. Microwave in 30-second intervals, stirring in between, until chocolate is melted and smooth.
4. Dip each strawberry into the melted chocolate, allowing excess chocolate to drip off.
5. Place the chocolate-covered strawberries on the prepared baking sheet.
6. Refrigerate for at least 30 minutes or until chocolate is set.
7. Serve chilled as a decadent and satisfying dessert option.

Baked Cinnamon Apple Chips:

- Ingredients:

1. 2 medium apples, cored
   and thinly sliced
2. 1 teaspoon ground
   cinnamon
3. 1 tablespoon granulated
   sweetener of choice

- Instructions:
  1. Preheat oven to 200°F
     (95°C) and line a baking
     sheet with parchment
     paper.
  2. In a bowl, toss apple slices
     with ground cinnamon
     and granulated sweetener
     until evenly coated.
  3. Arrange apple slices in a
     single layer on the
     prepared baking sheet.
  4. Bake in the preheated
     oven for 1.5 to 2 hours,
     flipping halfway through,
     or until apples are dried
     and crispy.

5. Remove from oven and let cool completely.

6. Serve as a crunchy and naturally sweet snack or dessert option.

Banana-Oat Cookies:

- Ingredients:
    1. 2 ripe bananas, mashed
    2. 1 cup old-fashioned oats
    3. 1/4 cup unsweetened applesauce
    4. 1/4 cup raisins or dried cranberries (optional)
    5. 1/4 teaspoon ground cinnamon
    6. 1/4 teaspoon vanilla extract
- Instructions:
    1. Preheat oven to 350°F (175°C) and line a baking sheet with parchment paper.

2. In a bowl, combine mashed bananas, oats, applesauce, raisins or dried cranberries (if using), ground cinnamon, and vanilla extract. Mix well.
3. Drop spoonfuls of the mixture onto the prepared baking sheet, forming cookies.
4. Bake for 15-20 minutes, or until cookies are golden brown and set.
5. Let cool before serving. These cookies are naturally sweet and make a great guilt-free treat.

Watermelon Sorbet:

- Ingredients:
  1. 4 cups seedless watermelon, cubed

2. 2 tablespoons fresh lime juice

3. 2 tablespoons honey or agave syrup

- Instructions:

1. Place the cubed watermelon on a baking sheet lined with parchment paper.

2. Freeze the watermelon cubes for at least 2 hours or until frozen solid.

3. Once frozen, transfer the watermelon cubes to a blender or food processor.

4. Add lime juice and honey or agave syrup to the blender.

5. Blend until smooth and creamy, scraping down the sides as needed.

6. Transfer the mixture to a shallow container and

freeze for another hour to
firm up.

7. Serve scoops of the
watermelon sorbet in
bowls or cones for a
refreshing and low-calorie
dessert.

Chocolate Chia Pudding:

- Ingredients:
    1. 2 tablespoons chia seeds
    2. 1 cup unsweetened almond
       milk (or any milk of
       choice)
    3. 1 tablespoon unsweetened
       cocoa powder
    4. 1 tablespoon maple syrup
       or honey
    5. 1/4 teaspoon vanilla
       extract
- Instructions:
    1. In a bowl or jar, combine
       chia seeds, almond milk,
       cocoa powder, maple

syrup or honey, and vanilla extract. Mix well.

2. Cover and refrigerate the mixture for at least 2 hours or overnight, stirring occasionally, until thickened.

3. Serve the chocolate chia pudding topped with fresh berries or sliced bananas for a nutritious and satisfying dessert option.

Baked Cinnamon Banana Chips:

- Ingredients:
    1. 2 ripe bananas, thinly sliced
    2. 1 tablespoon lemon juice
    3. 1 teaspoon ground cinnamon
- Instructions:
    1. Preheat oven to 200°F (95°C) and line a baking

sheet with parchment paper.

2. In a bowl, toss banana slices with lemon juice and ground cinnamon until evenly coated.

3. Arrange banana slices in a single layer on the prepared baking sheet.

4. Bake for 1.5 to 2 hours, flipping halfway through, or until banana chips are dried and crispy.

5. Let cool before serving. Enjoy these naturally sweet and crunchy chips as a healthy snack or dessert option.

Frozen Yogurt Berry Bites:

- Ingredients:
    1. 1 cup non-fat Greek yogurt
    2. 1 tablespoon honey or maple syrup

3. 1/2 cup mixed berries (such as raspberries, blueberries, and strawberries), chopped

- Instructions:
    1. In a bowl, mix together Greek yogurt and honey or maple syrup until well combined.
    2. Spoon the yogurt mixture into silicone ice cube molds, filling each mold halfway.
    3. Sprinkle chopped mixed berries over the yogurt mixture in each mold.
    4. Top with the remaining yogurt mixture, covering the berries.
    5. Insert toothpicks or small sticks into each mold.
    6. Freeze for at least 4 hours or until firm.
    7. Once frozen, remove the yogurt berry bites from the molds and serve immediately as a refreshing and low-calorie dessert option.

No-Bake Peanut Butter Energy Bites:

- Ingredients:
  1. 1 cup old-fashioned oats
  2. 1/2 cup natural peanut butter
  3. 1/4 cup honey
  4. 1/4 cup mini chocolate chips
  5. 1/4 cup ground flaxseed
  6. 1 teaspoon vanilla extract
- Instructions:
  1. In a bowl, mix together oats, peanut butter, honey, mini chocolate chips, ground flaxseed, and vanilla extract until well combined.
  2. Roll the mixture into small balls, about 1 inch in diameter.
  3. Place the energy bites on a parchment-lined baking sheet.
  4. Refrigerate for at least 30 minutes to firm up.
  5. Once firm, transfer the energy bites to an airtight container and store in the refrigerator.

6. Serve chilled as a satisfying and energizing snack or dessert option.

Chia Seed Pudding with Mango Puree:

- Ingredients:
    1. 1/4 cup chia seeds
    2. 1 cup unsweetened almond milk (or any milk of choice)
    3. 1 tablespoon honey or maple syrup
    4. 1 ripe mango, peeled and diced
    5. 1/4 cup water
- Instructions:
    1. In a bowl or jar, combine chia seeds, almond milk, and honey or maple syrup. Mix well.
    2. Cover and refrigerate the mixture for at least 2 hours or overnight, stirring occasionally, until thickened.
    3. In a blender, puree diced mango with water until smooth.

4. To serve, layer the chia seed pudding and mango puree in glasses or bowls.

5. Garnish with additional diced mango, if desired.

6. Serve chilled as a nutritious and naturally sweet dessert option.

Berry Frozen Yogurt Popsicles:

- Ingredients:
  1. 1 cup non-fat Greek yogurt
  2. 1 tablespoon honey or maple syrup
  3. 1 cup mixed berries (such as strawberries, blueberries, and raspberries), chopped

- Instructions:
  1. In a bowl, mix together Greek yogurt and honey or maple syrup until well combined.
  2. Stir in chopped mixed berries until evenly distributed.
  3. Pour the mixture into popsicle molds.

4. Insert popsicle sticks into the molds.

5. Freeze for at least 4 hours or until completely frozen.

6. Once frozen, remove the popsicles from the molds and serve immediately. Enjoy these fruity and creamy treats as a refreshing dessert option.

Chapter 10: SOUPS AND STEWS RECIPES

Vegetable Lentil Soup:

- Ingredients:
    1. 1 tablespoon olive oil
    2. 1 onion, chopped
    3. 2 carrots, diced
    4. 2 celery stalks, diced
    5. 2 garlic cloves, minced
    6. 1 cup dried lentils, rinsed

7. 4 cups low-sodium vegetable broth
8. 1 (14.5 oz) can diced tomatoes
9. 1 teaspoon dried thyme
10. Salt and pepper to taste
- Instructions:
    1. Heat olive oil in a large pot over medium heat.
    2. Add chopped onion, diced carrots, diced celery, and minced garlic. Cook until vegetables are softened, about 5 minutes.
    3. Add rinsed lentils, vegetable broth, diced tomatoes (with juices), and dried thyme to the pot.
    4. Bring the mixture to a boil, then reduce heat to low and simmer, covered, for 20-25 minutes or until lentils are tender.

5. Season with salt and pepper to taste.
6. Serve hot.

Chicken and Vegetable Quinoa Soup:

- Ingredients:
    1. 1 tablespoon olive oil
    2. 1 onion, chopped
    3. 2 carrots, diced
    4. 2 celery stalks, diced
    5. 2 cloves garlic, minced
    6. 6 cups low-sodium chicken broth
    7. 1 cup cooked quinoa
    8. 2 cups cooked shredded chicken breast
    9. 1 teaspoon dried thyme
    10. Salt and pepper to taste
- Instructions:
    1. Heat olive oil in a large pot over medium heat.
    2. Add chopped onion, diced carrots, diced celery, and minced garlic. Cook until

vegetables are softened, about 5 minutes.
3. Add low-sodium chicken broth, cooked quinoa, cooked shredded chicken breast, and dried thyme to the pot.
4. Bring the mixture to a boil, then reduce heat to low and simmer, covered, for 15-20 minutes.
5. Season with salt and pepper to taste.
6. Serve hot.

Turkey and Vegetable Chili:

- Ingredients:
    1. 1 tablespoon olive oil
    2. 1 onion, chopped
    3. 1 bell pepper, diced
    4. 2 cloves garlic, minced
    5. 1 pound lean ground turkey

6. 1 (15 oz) can kidney beans, drained and rinsed
7. 1 (15 oz) can diced tomatoes
8. 1 cup low-sodium chicken broth
9. 2 tablespoons chili powder
10. 1 teaspoon ground cumin
11. Salt and pepper to taste
- Instructions:
  1. Heat olive oil in a large pot over medium heat.
  2. Add chopped onion, diced bell pepper, and minced garlic. Cook until vegetables are softened, about 5 minutes.
  3. Add lean ground turkey to the pot and cook until browned, breaking it up with a spoon.
  4. Stir in drained and rinsed kidney beans, diced

tomatoes (with juices), low-sodium chicken broth, chili powder, and ground cumin.

5. Bring the mixture to a boil, then reduce heat to low and simmer, covered, for 20-25 minutes.
6. Season with salt and pepper to taste.
7. Serve hot.

Butternut Squash and Apple Soup:

- ○ Ingredients:
    1. 1 tablespoon olive oil
    2. 1 onion, chopped
    3. 1 butternut squash, peeled, seeded, and diced
    4. 2 apples, peeled, cored, and diced
    5. 4 cups low-sodium vegetable broth
    6. 1 teaspoon dried thyme
    7. Salt and pepper to taste

- Instructions:
    1. Heat olive oil in a large pot over medium heat.
    2. Add chopped onion and cook until softened, about 5 minutes.
    3. Add diced butternut squash, diced apples, low-sodium vegetable broth, and dried thyme to the pot.
    4. Bring the mixture to a boil, then reduce heat to low and simmer, covered, for 20-25 minutes or until butternut squash is tender.
    5. Use an immersion blender to puree the soup until smooth. Alternatively, carefully transfer the soup in batches to a blender and blend until smooth.
    6. Season with salt and pepper to taste.

7. Serve hot.

Minestrone Soup:

- Ingredients:
    1. 1 tablespoon olive oil
    2. 1 onion, diced
    3. 2 carrots, diced
    4. 2 celery stalks, diced
    5. 2 cloves garlic, minced
    6. 1 zucchini, diced
    7. 1 cup green beans, chopped
    8. 1 (14.5 oz) can diced tomatoes
    9. 4 cups low-sodium vegetable broth
    10. 1 teaspoon dried basil
    11. 1 teaspoon dried oregano
    12. 1/2 cup small pasta (such as ditalini or small shells)
    13. Salt and pepper to taste
- Instructions:
    1. Heat olive oil in a large pot over medium heat.

2. Add diced onion, carrots, celery, and minced garlic. Cook until vegetables are softened, about 5 minutes.
3. Add diced zucchini, chopped green beans, diced tomatoes (with juices), low-sodium vegetable broth, dried basil, and dried oregano to the pot.
4. Bring the mixture to a boil, then reduce heat to low and simmer, covered, for 15-20 minutes.
5. Stir in small pasta and continue to simmer for an additional 10-12 minutes or until pasta is cooked.
6. Season with salt and pepper to taste.
7. Serve hot, optionally garnished with grated Parmesan cheese.

Black Bean Soup:

- Ingredients:
    1. 1 tablespoon olive oil
    2. 1 onion, chopped
    3. 2 cloves garlic, minced
    4. 2 teaspoons ground cumin
    5. 1 teaspoon chili powder
    6. 2 (15 oz) cans black beans, drained and rinsed
    7. 4 cups low-sodium vegetable broth
    8. 1 (14.5 oz) can diced tomatoes
    9. Juice of 1 lime
    10. Salt and pepper to taste
    11. Fresh cilantro, chopped, for garnish (optional)
- Instructions:
    1. Heat olive oil in a large pot over medium heat.
    2. Add chopped onion and cook until softened, about 5 minutes.

3. Add minced garlic, ground cumin, and chili powder. Cook for an additional 1-2 minutes until fragrant.
4. Stir in drained and rinsed black beans, low-sodium vegetable broth, and diced tomatoes (with juices).
5. Bring the mixture to a boil, then reduce heat to low and simmer, covered, for 15-20 minutes.
6. Use an immersion blender to partially blend the soup until desired consistency is reached, leaving some beans whole.
7. Stir in lime juice and season with salt and pepper to taste.
8. Serve hot, garnished with fresh cilantro if desired.

Turkey and Vegetable Soup:

- Ingredients:
    1. 1 tablespoon olive oil
    2. 1 onion, chopped
    3. 2 carrots, diced
    4. 2 celery stalks, diced
    5. 2 cloves garlic, minced
    6. 1 pound lean ground turkey
    7. 4 cups low-sodium chicken broth
    8. 1 (14.5 oz) can diced tomatoes
    9. 1 teaspoon dried thyme
    10. Salt and pepper to taste
- Instructions:
    1. Heat olive oil in a large pot over medium heat.
    2. Add chopped onion, diced carrots, diced celery, and minced garlic. Cook until vegetables are softened, about 5 minutes.

3. Add lean ground turkey to
   the pot and cook until
   browned, breaking it up
   with a spoon.
4. Stir in low-sodium chicken
   broth, diced tomatoes
   (with juices), and dried
   thyme.
5. Bring the mixture to a boil,
   then reduce heat to low
   and simmer, covered, for
   15-20 minutes.
6. Season with salt and
   pepper to taste.
7. Serve hot.

Chunky Vegetable Stew:

- Ingredients:
  1. 1 tablespoon olive oil
  2. 1 onion, diced
  3. 2 carrots, diced
  4. 2 celery stalks, diced
  5. 2 cloves garlic, minced

6. 1 sweet potato, peeled and diced
7. 2 cups diced butternut squash
8. 4 cups low-sodium vegetable broth
9. 1 teaspoon dried thyme
10. Salt and pepper to taste

- Instructions:
    1. Heat olive oil in a large pot over medium heat.
    2. Add diced onion, carrots, celery, and minced garlic. Cook until vegetables are softened, about 5 minutes.
    3. Add diced sweet potato, diced butternut squash, low-sodium vegetable broth, and dried thyme to the pot.
    4. Bring the mixture to a boil, then reduce heat to low and simmer, covered, for

20-25 minutes or until vegetables are tender.
5. Season with salt and pepper to taste.
6. Serve hot.

Tomato Basil Soup:

- Ingredients:
    1. 1 tablespoon olive oil
    2. 1 onion, chopped
    3. 2 cloves garlic, minced
    4. 2 (14.5 oz) cans diced tomatoes
    5. 2 cups low-sodium vegetable broth
    6. 1 teaspoon dried basil
    7. Salt and pepper to taste
    8. Fresh basil leaves, chopped, for garnish (optional)
- Instructions:
    1. Heat olive oil in a large pot over medium heat.

2. Add chopped onion and cook until softened, about 5 minutes.
3. Add minced garlic and cook for an additional minute.
4. Stir in diced tomatoes (with juices), low-sodium vegetable broth, and dried basil.
5. Bring the mixture to a boil, then reduce heat to low and simmer, covered, for 20-25 minutes.
6. Use an immersion blender to puree the soup until smooth. Alternatively, carefully transfer the soup in batches to a blender and blend until smooth.
7. Season with salt and pepper to taste.

8. Serve hot, garnished with chopped fresh basil leaves if desired.

Chicken and Wild Rice Soup:

- Ingredients:
    1. 1 tablespoon olive oil
    2. 1 onion, chopped
    3. 2 carrots, diced
    4. 2 celery stalks, diced
    5. 2 cloves garlic, minced
    6. 6 cups low-sodium chicken broth
    7. 1 cup cooked wild rice
    8. 2 cups cooked shredded chicken breast
    9. 1 teaspoon dried thyme
    10. Salt and pepper to taste
- Instructions:
    1. Heat olive oil in a large pot over medium heat.
    2. Add chopped onion, diced carrots, diced celery, and minced garlic. Cook until

vegetables are softened, about 5 minutes.
3. Add low-sodium chicken broth to the pot and bring to a boil.
4. Stir in cooked wild rice, cooked shredded chicken breast, and dried thyme.
5. Reduce heat to low and simmer, covered, for 15-20 minutes.
6. Season with salt and pepper to taste.
7. Serve hot.

Vegetarian Black Bean Stew:

- Ingredients:
  1. 1 tablespoon olive oil
  2. 1 onion, chopped
  3. 2 cloves garlic, minced
  4. 2 bell peppers (any color), diced
  5. 2 carrots, diced
  6. 2 celery stalks, diced

7. 2 (15 oz) cans black beans, drained and rinsed

8. 1 (14.5 oz) can diced tomatoes

9. 2 cups low-sodium vegetable broth

10. 1 teaspoon ground cumin

11. 1 teaspoon chili powder

12. Salt and pepper to taste

13. Fresh cilantro, chopped, for garnish (optional)

- Instructions:

1. Heat olive oil in a large pot over medium heat.

2. Add chopped onion and minced garlic. Cook until softened, about 5 minutes.

3. Add diced bell peppers, diced carrots, and diced celery. Cook for an additional 5 minutes.

4. Stir in drained and rinsed black beans, diced

tomatoes (with juices), low-sodium vegetable broth, ground cumin, and chili powder.
5. Bring the mixture to a boil, then reduce heat to low and simmer, covered, for 20-25 minutes.
6. Season with salt and pepper to taste.
7. Serve hot, garnished with chopped fresh cilantro if desired.

Creamy Cauliflower Soup:

- Ingredients:
    1. 1 tablespoon olive oil
    2. 1 onion, chopped
    3. 2 cloves garlic, minced
    4. 1 head cauliflower, chopped into florets
    5. 4 cups low-sodium vegetable broth

6. 1/2 cup unsweetened almond milk
7. Salt and pepper to taste
8. Fresh chives, chopped, for garnish (optional)

- Instructions:
  1. Heat olive oil in a large pot over medium heat.
  2. Add chopped onion and minced garlic. Cook until softened, about 5 minutes.
  3. Add chopped cauliflower florets and low-sodium vegetable broth to the pot. Bring to a boil.
  4. Reduce heat to low and simmer, covered, for 20-25 minutes or until cauliflower is tender.
  5. Use an immersion blender to puree the soup until smooth. Alternatively, carefully transfer the soup

in batches to a blender and blend until smooth.

6. Stir in unsweetened almond milk and season with salt and pepper to taste.
7. Serve hot, garnished with chopped fresh chives if desired.

Sweet Potato and Lentil Stew:

- Ingredients:
    1. 1 tablespoon olive oil
    2. 1 onion, diced
    3. 2 cloves garlic, minced
    4. 2 sweet potatoes, peeled and diced
    5. 1 cup dried lentils, rinsed
    6. 4 cups low-sodium vegetable broth
    7. 1 (14.5 oz) can diced tomatoes
    8. 1 teaspoon ground cumin
    9. 1 teaspoon smoked paprika
    10. Salt and pepper to taste

- Instructions:
  1. Heat olive oil in a large pot over medium heat.
  2. Add diced onion and minced garlic. Cook until softened, about 5 minutes.
  3. Add diced sweet potatoes, rinsed lentils, low-sodium vegetable broth, diced tomatoes (with juices), ground cumin, and smoked paprika to the pot.
  4. Bring the mixture to a boil, then reduce heat to low and simmer, covered, for 25-30 minutes or until sweet potatoes and lentils are tender.
  5. Season with salt and pepper to taste.
  6. Serve hot.

Spinach and White Bean Soup:

- Ingredients:
  1. 1 tablespoon olive oil
  2. 1 onion, diced

3. 2 cloves garlic, minced
4. 4 cups low-sodium vegetable broth
5. 1 (14.5 oz) can diced tomatoes
6. 1 (15 oz) can white beans, drained and rinsed
7. 4 cups fresh spinach leaves
8. 1 teaspoon dried Italian seasoning
9. Salt and pepper to taste

- Instructions:
    1. Heat olive oil in a large pot over medium heat.
    2. Add diced onion and minced garlic. Cook until softened, about 5 minutes.
    3. Add low-sodium vegetable broth, diced tomatoes (with juices), drained and rinsed white beans, and dried Italian seasoning to the pot.
    4. Bring the mixture to a boil, then reduce heat to low and simmer, covered, for 15-20 minutes.

5. Stir in fresh spinach leaves and continue to simmer for an additional 5 minutes or until spinach is wilted.
6. Season with salt and pepper to taste.
7. Serve hot.

Chicken Tortilla Soup:

- Ingredients:
    1. 1 tablespoon olive oil
    2. 1 onion, diced
    3. 2 cloves garlic, minced
    4. 1 bell pepper, diced
    5. 1 jalapeño pepper, seeded and diced
    6. 1 teaspoon ground cumin
    7. 1 teaspoon chili powder
    8. 4 cups low-sodium chicken broth
    9. 1 (14.5 oz) can diced tomatoes
    10. 1 cup cooked shredded chicken breast
    11. Juice of 1 lime

12. Salt and pepper to taste
13. Tortilla strips, for garnish (optional)

- Instructions:
    1. Heat olive oil in a large pot over medium heat.
    2. Add diced onion, minced garlic, diced bell pepper, and diced jalapeño pepper. Cook until softened, about 5 minutes.
    3. Stir in ground cumin and chili powder. Cook for an additional minute.
    4. Add low-sodium chicken broth, diced tomatoes (with juices), and cooked shredded chicken breast to the pot.
    5. Bring the mixture to a boil, then reduce heat to low and simmer, covered, for 15-20 minutes.
    6. Stir in lime juice and season with salt and pepper to taste.
    7. Serve hot, garnished with tortilla strips if desired.

Creamy Mushroom Soup:

- Ingredients:
    1. 1 tablespoon olive oil
    2. 1 onion, diced
    3. 2 cloves garlic, minced
    4. 16 oz mushrooms, sliced
    5. 4 cups low-sodium vegetable broth
    6. 1 tablespoon cornstarch (or flour)
    7. 1 cup unsweetened almond milk
    8. 1 teaspoon dried thyme
    9. Salt and pepper to taste
- Instructions:
    1. Heat olive oil in a large pot over medium heat.
    2. Add diced onion and minced garlic. Cook until softened, about 5 minutes.
    3. Add sliced mushrooms to the pot and cook until they release their moisture and become tender, about 5-7 minutes.

4. In a small bowl, whisk together cornstarch (or flour) and unsweetened almond milk until smooth.
5. Pour the almond milk mixture into the pot, stirring constantly.
6. Stir in low-sodium vegetable broth and dried thyme.
7. Bring the mixture to a simmer and cook for an additional 10-15 minutes, stirring occasionally, until slightly thickened.
8. Season with salt and pepper to taste.
9. Serve hot.

28DAY MEAL PLAN

Day 1:

- Breakfast: Greek yogurt parfait with mixed berries and a sprinkle of granola (5 SmartPoints)
- Lunch: Turkey and vegetable wrap with whole wheat tortilla, turkey slices, lettuce, tomato, and mustard (6 SmartPoints)
- Dinner: Baked lemon herb salmon with steamed broccoli and quinoa (9 SmartPoints)
- Snack: Apple slices with a tablespoon of almond butter (4 SmartPoints)

Day 2:

- Breakfast: Veggie omelet made with egg whites, spinach, tomatoes, and mushrooms (3 SmartPoints)
- Lunch: Chickpea salad with mixed greens, cherry tomatoes, cucumber, bell peppers, and balsamic vinaigrette dressing (5 SmartPoints)

- Dinner: Grilled chicken breast with roasted sweet potatoes and green beans (8 SmartPoints)
- Snack: Carrot sticks with hummus (3 SmartPoints)

Day 3:

- Breakfast: Oatmeal topped with sliced banana and a drizzle of honey (5 SmartPoints)
- Lunch: Quinoa salad with black beans, corn, diced avocado, cherry tomatoes, and lime-cilantro dressing (7 SmartPoints)
- Dinner: Spaghetti squash with marinara sauce and lean ground turkey (8 SmartPoints)
- Snack: Low-fat string cheese with whole grain crackers (3 SmartPoints)

Day 4:

- Breakfast: Whole wheat toast with avocado mash and poached eggs (6 SmartPoints)
- Lunch: Lentil soup with a side salad of mixed greens, carrots, and vinaigrette dressing (6 SmartPoints)
- Dinner: Stir-fried tofu with mixed vegetables served over brown rice (7 SmartPoints)
- Snack: Greek yogurt with a sprinkle of cinnamon and sliced strawberries (3 SmartPoints)

Day 5:

- Breakfast: Smoothie made with spinach, banana, unsweetened almond milk, and protein powder (4 SmartPoints)
- Lunch: Turkey and vegetable stir-fry with broccoli, bell peppers, snap peas,

and teriyaki sauce, served over cauliflower rice (6 SmartPoints)
- Dinner: Grilled shrimp skewers with quinoa tabbouleh salad (9 SmartPoints)
- Snack: Cottage cheese with pineapple chunks (3 SmartPoints)

Day 6:

- Breakfast: Whole grain cereal with skim milk and sliced strawberries (5 SmartPoints)
- Lunch: Turkey and cranberry wrap with whole wheat tortilla, sliced turkey breast, spinach, cranberry sauce, and light mayo (7 SmartPoints)
- Dinner: Baked chicken breast with roasted Brussels sprouts and a small sweet potato (8 SmartPoints)
- Snack: Edamame (steamed soybeans) with a sprinkle of sea salt (2 SmartPoints)

Day 7:

- Breakfast: Egg muffins with spinach, tomatoes, and feta cheese (3 SmartPoints)
- Lunch: Quinoa and black bean stuffed bell peppers with a side salad of mixed greens and vinaigrette dressing (7 SmartPoints)
- Dinner: Vegetarian chili made with beans, tomatoes, corn, and bell peppers, served with a side of whole grain bread (8 SmartPoints)
- Snack: Sliced cucumber with tzatziki sauce (2 SmartPoints)

Day 8:

- Breakfast: Whole grain toast topped with mashed avocado and sliced hard-boiled egg (6 SmartPoints)
- Lunch: Turkey and cranberry wrap with whole wheat tortilla, sliced turkey

breast, spinach, cranberry sauce, and light mayo (7 SmartPoints)
- Dinner: Grilled salmon with roasted asparagus and quinoa (9 SmartPoints)
- Snack: Air-popped popcorn (3 SmartPoints)

Day 9:

- Breakfast: Greek yogurt parfait with mixed berries and a sprinkle of granola (5 SmartPoints)
- Lunch: Lentil soup with a side salad of mixed greens, cherry tomatoes, and balsamic vinaigrette dressing (6 SmartPoints)
- Dinner: Chicken fajita bowls with grilled chicken breast, sautéed bell peppers and onions, black beans, brown rice, and salsa (8 SmartPoints)
- Snack: Apple slices with a tablespoon of peanut butter (4 SmartPoints)

Day 10:

- Breakfast: Spinach and mushroom omelet made with egg whites (3 SmartPoints)
- Lunch: Quinoa salad with black beans, corn, diced avocado, cherry tomatoes, and lime-cilantro dressing (7 SmartPoints)
- Dinner: Turkey meatballs with marinara sauce over zucchini noodles (8 SmartPoints)
- Snack: Low-fat yogurt with a sprinkle of cinnamon and sliced bananas (3 SmartPoints)

Day 11:

- Breakfast: Oatmeal topped with sliced banana and a drizzle of honey (5 SmartPoints)
- Lunch: Chicken Caesar salad with grilled chicken breast, romaine lettuce, cherry tomatoes, Parmesan

cheese, and Caesar dressing (8 SmartPoints)

- Dinner: Beef and vegetable stir-fry with broccoli, snap peas, carrots, and teriyaki sauce, served over brown rice (9 SmartPoints)
- Snack: Carrot sticks with hummus (3 SmartPoints)

Day 12:

- Breakfast: Whole wheat toast with mashed avocado and poached eggs (6 SmartPoints)
- Lunch: Caprese salad with sliced tomatoes, fresh mozzarella, basil leaves, balsamic glaze, and a drizzle of olive oil (6 SmartPoints)
- Dinner: Baked cod with roasted Brussels sprouts and quinoa (8 SmartPoints)
- Snack: Cottage cheese with pineapple chunks (3 SmartPoints)

Day 13:

- Breakfast: Smoothie made with spinach, banana, unsweetened almond milk, and protein powder (4 SmartPoints)
- Lunch: Turkey and vegetable wrap with whole wheat tortilla, turkey slices, lettuce, tomato, and mustard (6 SmartPoints)
- Dinner: Vegetarian stuffed bell peppers with a side salad of mixed greens and vinaigrette dressing (7 SmartPoints)
- Snack: Edamame (steamed soybeans) with a sprinkle of sea salt (2 SmartPoints)

Day 14:

- Breakfast: Egg muffins with spinach, tomatoes, and feta cheese (3 SmartPoints)

- Lunch: Turkey and avocado salad with mixed greens, sliced turkey breast, diced avocado, cherry tomatoes, and balsamic vinaigrette dressing (6 SmartPoints)
- Dinner: Spaghetti squash with marinara sauce and lean ground turkey (8 SmartPoints)
- Snack: Low-fat string cheese with whole grain crackers (3 SmartPoints)

Day 15:

- Breakfast: Greek yogurt parfait with mixed berries and a sprinkle of granola (5 SmartPoints)
- Lunch: Turkey and cranberry wrap with whole wheat tortilla, sliced turkey breast, spinach, cranberry sauce, and light mayo (7 SmartPoints)
- Dinner: Grilled salmon with roasted asparagus and quinoa (9 SmartPoints)

- Snack: Air-popped popcorn (3 SmartPoints)

Day 16:

- Breakfast: Spinach and mushroom omelet made with egg whites (3 SmartPoints)
- Lunch: Lentil soup with a side salad of mixed greens, cherry tomatoes, and balsamic vinaigrette dressing (6 SmartPoints)
- Dinner: Chicken fajita bowls with grilled chicken breast, sautéed bell peppers and onions, black beans, brown rice, and salsa (8 SmartPoints)
- Snack: Apple slices with a tablespoon of peanut butter (4 SmartPoints)

Day 17:

- Breakfast: Oatmeal topped with sliced banana and a drizzle of honey (5 SmartPoints)

- Lunch: Quinoa salad with black beans, corn, diced avocado, cherry tomatoes, and lime-cilantro dressing (7 SmartPoints)
- Dinner: Turkey meatballs with marinara sauce over zucchini noodles (8 SmartPoints)
- Snack: Low-fat yogurt with a sprinkle of cinnamon and sliced bananas (3 SmartPoints)

Day 18:

- Breakfast: Whole wheat toast with mashed avocado and poached eggs (6 SmartPoints)
- Lunch: Chicken Caesar salad with grilled chicken breast, romaine lettuce, cherry tomatoes, Parmesan cheese, and Caesar dressing (8 SmartPoints)
- Dinner: Beef and vegetable stir-fry with broccoli, snap peas, carrots, and

teriyaki sauce, served over brown rice (9 SmartPoints)

- Snack: Carrot sticks with hummus (3 SmartPoints)

Day 19:

- Breakfast: Smoothie made with spinach, banana, unsweetened almond milk, and protein powder (4 SmartPoints)
- Lunch: Turkey and vegetable wrap with whole wheat tortilla, turkey slices, lettuce, tomato, and mustard (6 SmartPoints)
- Dinner: Vegetarian stuffed bell peppers with a side salad of mixed greens and vinaigrette dressing (7 SmartPoints)
- Snack: Edamame (steamed soybeans) with a sprinkle of sea salt (2 SmartPoints)

Day 20:

- Breakfast: Egg muffins with spinach, tomatoes, and feta cheese (3 SmartPoints)
- Lunch: Turkey and avocado salad with mixed greens, sliced turkey breast, diced avocado, cherry tomatoes, and balsamic vinaigrette dressing (6 SmartPoints)
- Dinner: Spaghetti squash with marinara sauce and lean ground turkey (8 SmartPoints)
- Snack: Low-fat string cheese with whole grain crackers (3 SmartPoints)

Day 21:

- Breakfast: Greek yogurt parfait with mixed berries and a sprinkle of granola (5 SmartPoints)
- Lunch: Turkey and cranberry wrap with whole wheat tortilla, sliced turkey

breast, spinach, cranberry sauce, and light mayo (7 SmartPoints)
- Dinner: Grilled salmon with roasted asparagus and quinoa (9 SmartPoints)
- Snack: Air-popped popcorn (3 SmartPoints)

Day 22:

- Breakfast: Whole grain toast topped with mashed avocado and sliced hard-boiled egg (6 SmartPoints)
- Lunch: Lentil soup with a side salad of mixed greens, cherry tomatoes, and balsamic vinaigrette dressing (6 SmartPoints)
- Dinner: Grilled chicken breast with roasted Brussels sprouts and quinoa (8 SmartPoints)
- Snack: Carrot sticks with hummus (3 SmartPoints)

Day 23:

- Breakfast: Greek yogurt parfait with mixed berries and a sprinkle of granola (5 SmartPoints)
- Lunch: Turkey and vegetable stir-fry with broccoli, bell peppers, snap peas, and teriyaki sauce, served over cauliflower rice (6 SmartPoints)
- Dinner: Baked cod with roasted asparagus and brown rice (8 SmartPoints)
- Snack: Low-fat yogurt with a sprinkle of cinnamon and sliced bananas (3 SmartPoints)

Day 24:

- Breakfast: Spinach and mushroom omelet made with egg whites (3 SmartPoints)
- Lunch: Chickpea salad with mixed greens, cherry tomatoes, cucumber,

bell peppers, and balsamic vinaigrette dressing (5 SmartPoints)

- Dinner: Turkey chili with mixed beans, diced tomatoes, and chili seasoning, served with a side of whole grain bread (7 SmartPoints)
- Snack: Apple slices with a tablespoon of peanut butter (4 SmartPoints)

Day 25:

- Breakfast: Oatmeal topped with sliced banana and a drizzle of honey (5 SmartPoints)
- Lunch: Turkey and cranberry wrap with whole wheat tortilla, sliced turkey breast, spinach, cranberry sauce, and light mayo (7 SmartPoints)
- Dinner: Grilled shrimp skewers with quinoa tabbouleh salad (9 SmartPoints)
- Snack: Air-popped popcorn (3 SmartPoints)

Day 26:

- Breakfast: Smoothie made with spinach, banana, unsweetened almond milk, and protein powder (4 SmartPoints)
- Lunch: Caprese salad with sliced tomatoes, fresh mozzarella, basil leaves, balsamic glaze, and a drizzle of olive oil (6 SmartPoints)
- Dinner: Vegetarian stuffed bell peppers with a side salad of mixed greens and vinaigrette dressing (7 SmartPoints)
- Snack: Edamame (steamed soybeans) with a sprinkle of sea salt (2 SmartPoints)

Day 27:

- Breakfast: Egg muffins with spinach, tomatoes, and feta cheese (3 SmartPoints)

- Lunch: Turkey and avocado salad with mixed greens, sliced turkey breast, diced avocado, cherry tomatoes, and balsamic vinaigrette dressing (6 SmartPoints)
- Dinner: Spaghetti squash with marinara sauce and lean ground turkey (8 SmartPoints)
- Snack: Low-fat string cheese with whole grain crackers (3 SmartPoints)

Day 28:

- Breakfast: Greek yogurt parfait with mixed berries and a sprinkle of granola (5 SmartPoints)
- Lunch: Turkey and cranberry wrap with whole wheat tortilla, sliced turkey breast, spinach, cranberry sauce, and light mayo (7 SmartPoints)
- Dinner: Grilled salmon with roasted asparagus and quinoa (9 SmartPoints)
- Snack: Air-popped popcorn (3 SmartPoints)

CONCLUSION

Congratulations on taking the first step towards a healthier, happier you! With the Weight Watchers Cookbook for Beginners, you've unlocked the secret to delicious and sustainable weight loss. Remember, every bite is a choice, and every choice is a chance to nourish your body and soul.

As you close this book, remember that weight loss is not just about numbers on the scale, but about the journey of self-love, self-care, and self-discovery. You've got this! You've got the tools, the recipes, and the support to achieve your goals.

So go ahead, indulge in the sweetness of success, and savor every moment of your weight loss journey. You are worthy of a healthy, happy, and delicious life. Bon appétit, and happy losing!"

This conclusion aims to:

- Congratulate the reader on taking the first step towards a healthier lifestyle
- Emphasize the importance of self-love and self-care in the weight loss journey
- Encourage the reader to embrace their journey and celebrate their successes
- Leave a lasting impression and motivate readers to buy the book

THE END